# Nursing Perspectives on Quality of Life

*Nursing Perspectives on Quality of Life* describes a new philosophical approach to a concept widely used in nursing practice. Peter Draper challenges existing definitions of quality of life, the methods used to measure it in different contexts and the impact of research findings on health policy.

Presenting new research into the quality of life of older people in hospital wards, the author argues that nurses need a model which more accurately reflects their patients' concerns and allows them to develop practical ways of promoting the well-being of people in their care.

Part One examines quantitative approaches to the quality of life, discussing social indicators, the Quality Adjusted Life Year (QALY), and medical outcomes literature. In Part Two the author proposes an alternative, qualitative approach to understanding the concept based on philosophical hermeneutics. Part Three presents original research into the quality of life of older people in hospital wards. Looking at what patients and carers consider to be important, such as personal possessions and clothing, the author considers what it means to respect a person's individuality and the impact this has on the organization of patient care.

Combining original research and a critical analysis of existing models, *Nursing Perspectives on Quality of Life* is suitable for students on undergraduate and postgraduate nursing courses.

**Peter Draper** is Lecturer in Nursing at the University of Hull.

**Routledge Essentials for Nurses** cover four key areas of nursing:

- core theoretical studies
- psychological and physical care
- nurse education
- new directions in nursing and health care

Written by experienced practitioners and teachers, books in this series encourage a critical approach to nursing concepts and show how research findings are relevant to nursing practice.

The series editors are **Robert Newell**, Lecturer in Nursing Studies, University of Hull and **David Thompson**, Professor of Nursing Studies, University of Hull.

Also in this series:

*Nursing Theories and Models* Hugh McKenna
*Teaching and Assessing Learners* Mary Chambers

# Nursing Perspectives on Quality of Life

Peter Draper

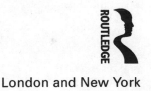

London and New York

First published 1997
by Routledge
11 New Fetter Lane, London EC4P 4EE

Simultaneously published in the USA and Canada
by Routledge
29 West 35th Street, New York, NY 10001

Typeset in Times by M Rules

Printed and bound in Great Britain by TJ Press International Ltd,
Padstow, Cornwall

*British Library Cataloguing in Publication Data*
A catalogue record for this book is available from the British Library

*Library of Congress Cataloguing in Publication Data*
Draper, Peter, 1957–
 Perspectives on quality of life / Peter Draper.
 p. cm. – (Routledge essentials for nurses)
 Includes bibliographical reference and index.
 1. Nursing – Philosophy. 2. Quality of life. 3. Nursing ethics.
I. Title. II. Series.
RT84.5.D73 1997
                              610.73'01 – dc21    96–36838
                                                    CIP

ISBN 0–415–14169–9
ISBN 0–415–14170–2 (pbk)

# Contents

# Tables

# Acknowledgements

The author and publisher would like to thank the following for their permission to include copyright material: Blackwell Publishers for an extract from Martin Heidegger (1962) *Being and Time*; BMJ Publishing Group for an extract from A. Williams (1985) 'The economics of coronary artery bypass grafting', *British Medical Journal* 291: 325–9. Every effort has been made to secure permission for the inclusion of other copyright material.

# Introduction

There is currently a great deal of interest in the concept of quality of life among health professionals. For instance, health economists suggest that information about the impact of treatment on patients' quality of life can enable scarce financial resources to be targeted in the most effective manner, and medical practitioners often publish research into the effect of individual methods of treatment on quality of life. There has, however, been rather less research from the nursing perspective into the usefulness of the concept.

This book has two aims. The first is to describe and evaluate two important bodies of research that relate quality of life to health: the quality adjusted life year (QALY), and evaluative medical research that takes quality of life as an outcome. This aim is achieved in three ways: by examining historical sources of quality of life research, by critical discussion of published work, and by teasing out the philosophical assumptions that are held by many researchers in the quality of life field. Part I addresses these issues. It concludes that most quality of life researchers are motivated by a desire to measure the concept, and that their work is underpinned by a positivist orientation to the social world.

The book's second aim is to explore some of the implications of the concept of quality of life for nursing practice – particularly the nursing care of older people who are resident in places other than their own homes, such as nursing homes and hospital wards. It is argued that the positivist orientation of medical research into quality of life reduces its significance for nurses who want to develop practical ways of promoting the quality of the lives of patients and clients, and it is suggested that this goal can most fruitfully be achieved if an alternative philosophical orientation is developed. Part II proposes that the study of philosophical hermeneutics offers a suitable basis for nursing research into the nature of quality of life, and its application to nursing care. Hermeneutics is briefly described, and the background to the author's quality of life research is discussed.

Part III presents the findings of an original research programme into the quality of life of older people in nursing homes. Chapter 9 discusses the significance of places, personal possessions and clothing; and Chapter 10 explores what it means to treat people as individuals and examines the effect of such treatment on their lives. Finally, the implications of the research for the organisation of nursing care are discussed.

PART I

# The concept of quality of life and its use in health research

# Chapter 1
# Introducing quality of life

There is considerable interest in the concept of quality of life among nurses, medical practitioners, researchers, health economists, and many other groups who work in and around the health services. Their interest reflects more general debates about the meaning and relevance of quality of life in fields as diverse as medical ethics, where the concept is related to arguments about euthanasia and abortion; environmental ethics; and moral issues in law such as crime and punishment. Politicians also frequently refer to the effect that their policies will have on the quality of the lives of their constituents and the nation at large. It is surprising that such a widely used concept, to which reference is made in the literature of so many academic disciplines, should be difficult to define in a satisfactory way; but the assumption with which this book begins is that the meaning of quality of life is vague. Indeed, many researchers in the field do not bother to discuss its meaning at all. In my view, the situation that exists today is similar to that described by McCall in 1980. McCall suggested that far from knowing what quality of life is, we do not even know what category of thing it is. He suggested that researchers are unable to decide whether it is a state of mind or a state of society, and are unclear as to whether its definition varies from person to person, from culture to culture, and from place to place. He also notes important differences of opinion about whether, and how, quality of life can be measured.

Generally speaking, it is useful to divide researchers in the quality of life field into two groups. Members of the first group subscribe to what can be called the 'social scientific' approach. They tend to regard quality of life as a rather concrete phenomenon which is present in people's lives to a greater or a lesser extent. They believe in principle that quality of life can be measured, and often expend considerable effort in designing and validating scales to be used for this purpose. Many people who take this approach also believe that it is possible to change the quality of people's lives (Romney *et al.* 1994). Medical practitioners, for instance, will argue that their treatments have a beneficial effect on their patients' quality of life, even when they make no discernible difference to patients' length of life; and they try to demonstrate this difference through evaluation research. In the same way, politicians will argue that the net effect of their policies is an increase in quality of life, and may fund social research in an attempt to show a sceptical electorate that this difference really exists.

The second group of researchers takes a very different, rather philosophical approach to quality of life. Their thinking can be traced back to the work of Aristotle, the ancient Greek philosopher. The writings of Aristotle contain the word '*eudaemonia*', which has often been translated as 'happiness' but which contemporary scholars tend to translate as 'human flourishing' (Den Uyl and Machan 1983). This approach to quality of life can be called 'eudaemonistic'. It is concerned with the nature of human beings and their social environment (Aiken 1982); and it seeks to identify conditions in which human beings can flourish.

Most of this book is roughly split between these two approaches. In Part I, we examine the social scientific approach in some detail. Because the literature in this field is so extensive, it is important to approach it in a way that is at once systematic and selective, so that important themes and debates can be identified. Three specific aspects are discussed: social indicators research (Chapter 2); the quality adjusted life year, or QALY (Chapter 3); and medical research which uses quality of life as an outcome in clinical trials (Chapter 4).

The social indicators literature is discussed because it represents probably the earliest systematic attempt to define and measure quality of life. It refers to a number of fundamental issues found throughout quality of life research, including the following:

● Should quality of life be regarded as a subjective or an objective phenomenon?
● Can quality of life be measured?

● Can the quality of people's lives be improved if the correct actions are taken?

QALYs and medical outcomes research both represent the application of quality of life to health. The QALY literature suggests that quality of life data can be used to inform resource allocation decisions in the health service, and examines the ethical issues created when this is done. The medical outcomes literature clearly illustrates some of the practical problems associated with the measurement of quality of life in the context of empirical research. Chapter 4 summarises a number of common themes that are found throughout the quality of life literature and discusses the relevance of the social scientific approach for nursing practice.

# Chapter 2
# Social indicators of quality of life

The social indicators movement is a good place to begin our examination of the social scientific approach to quality of life. This is because scholars working in social indicators research were the first to attempt to measure the concept and to map its attributes and distribution among the population. This literature describes a series of classic debates that characterise a great deal of quality of life research, as shown in Box 2.1.

---

**Box 2.1** Key debates in quality of life research

- whether quality of life is best seen as a subjective or an objective phenomenon;
- whether it is a characteristic of individual people or of populations;
- whether or not it is amenable to manipulation and change by a third party.

---

The first systematic quality of life research was probably conducted by the 'political arithmeticians', a group of mathematicians, chemists, naturalists and others from the natural scientific tradition who worked in the nineteenth century, and who became convinced that the intellectual tools of their scientific disciplines could be applied beneficially to some of the social problems that existed in their day. Although they would not have used or recognised the term 'quality of life', their work made possible a number of pioneering surveys of poverty in nineteenth-century England (Lazarsfeld 1961).

Modern research into social indicators of quality of life was also anticipated by Otto Neurath, a Marxist philosopher (Callebaut 1978). Neurath criticised the economists of his day for using vague and rather general terms such as 'the greatest good for the greatest number', 'the standard of living', 'the general welfare' and 'the good of the people' when evaluating the impact of economic policy on people's lives. He suggested that it ought to be possible to correlate people's social circumstances with an index of their standard of living, and then to investigate how the two are linked. In this way, he hoped that it would be possible to identify the economic 'inputs' that would lead to the desired 'output' of a good standard of living or quality of life. Neurath's work is remembered not for the impact that it had at its time, but because it has implications that are very familiar to modern quality of life researchers. Many quality of life researchers in medicine, nursing and the health-related disciplines believe that if you get the 'inputs' right by treating patients in a particular way, for instance, you can bring about the desired 'output' of a life of quality. A good deal of quality of life research is concerned with being able to measure the quality of life accurately and so to identify those treatments that are most effective in promoting it.

Neurath's ideas had little impact in his own day, but the attractive concept that it might be possible to quantify quality of life, and relate it as an outcome to public and economic policy, re-emerged in the 1960s. A social psychologist named Raymond Bauer then became interested in the impact that the NASA space programme was having on American society. In his preface to Bauer's book, Gross (1966) expressed many of the arguments which the social indicators movement was to take for granted.

Gross criticised American policy makers for over-emphasising conventional indicators of economic performance such as the gross national product (GNP). As Callebaut (1978) suggests, GNP is useful as a measure of economic activity, but it disregards the things that money cannot buy, and the quality of goods and services produced; and it does not take into account the social costs arising from production. Gross went on to criticise the emphasis that American policy makers were placing on cost-benefit analysis, and their assumption that all meaningful benefits from government

programmes could be expressed in dollars and cents. He proposed
a shift in emphasis from economy to society, suggesting that, for
many of the important topics on which social critics pass judgement, there are no yardsticks for measuring whether things are
getting better or worse.

Gross, like Neurath before him, appears to have been frustrated
by the economists' inability to measure inputs and outputs in a
clear way in order to relate economic and social policy to quality of
life; and once again, his attitude is reflected in modern quality of
life research in medicine, and its desire to measure the quality of life
with ever greater accuracy. This desire depends on various assumptions: that it can, in fact, be measured; and that the world is regular
and predictable to some degree. These and other assumptions will
be discussed in more detail below.

In America, President Johnson was sympathetic to arguments of
the kind that Gross put forward, and he established a Panel on
Social Indicators, consisting of social scientists and politicians, to
explore new approaches to social accounting (Moberg and Brusek
1978). In its first report, this panel argued that the American nation
had no comprehensive set of statistics to reflect social progress or
decline, and it noted that there was a marked discrepancy between
economic indicators, such as statistics on national income and retail
prices, and evidence of social discontent, such as increasing street
crime and the apparent alienation of young people. Social indicators were proposed as a way of monitoring the social condition of
the nation, so that politicians could make appropriate decisions
about economic and social policy.

It is important at this point to note that social indicators research
emerged from a political concern with certain social and economic
phenomena, and that social indicators themselves were designed to
be of use to politicians in the formulation of policy. This is significant because it is sometimes argued and more often assumed that
quality of life indicators of all kinds are essentially neutral, in that
they do not embody a particular ideology or set of beliefs. One of
the key aspects of the critique of the social scientific approach to
quality of life, outlined below, is that quality of life measurements
are never neutral, because the data they provide are invariably
employed in a political debate of some kind. Sometimes, as in the

case of social indicators, the outcome of this debate determines policy directions, while at other times the data are used as a basis for resource allocation decision. The political context of quality of life research often has a direct effect on the formulation of the indicators used to measure quality of life. This fact makes it difficult to sustain the view that measures of quality of life can ever be objective or 'value free'.

The early literature of social indicators of quality of life is often divided into two contrasting approaches: objective and subjective (Andrews 1974). Each of these is now discussed in more detail.

## Objective social indicators

The objectivists assumed there was a cause-and-effect relationship between quality of life, the consumption of public and market goods, and aspects of the physical environment. They advocated collating crime rates, population density figures and the level of public service provision, to give an 'objective' index of quality of life in a given population. This was the approach taken by Gehrmann (1978), who suggested that quality of life studies should concentrate on infrastructure facilities such as education, health and recreation, and those parts of the social domain which are 'measurable in objective terms'. He proposed to include data on crime, safety, social participation, social disintegration and unemployment. His work makes it easy to recognise one of the principal difficulties with this approach. Far from being objective, the measurement of many of these phenomena is highly contentious. The definition and measurement of unemployment, for instance, are matters not of objective fact but of political debate informed by ideological perspective.

Another researcher who took the objectivist approach is Liu (1975), whose work illustrates a number of further difficulties. Liu argued that the quality of life of an individual is the sum of a set of 'wants', whose satisfaction makes the individual happy. He considered that the things which make people happy can be placed into two groups: physical and spiritual. Physical things included quantifiable goods, services, material wealth, etc., while spiritual things included psychological, sociological and anthropological factors such as community belongingness, esteem, self-actualisation (see below), love and affection. Liu omitted the spiritual concerns from his approach to quality of life because he was unable to measure them, thereby ending up with a definition of quality of life restricted to a number of physical inputs consisting of social factors (individual status, individual equality, and living conditions); economic inputs (economic status, technological development and agricultural production); and political inputs (health and welfare provision, educational development and government).

Liu's approach contains a number of difficulties:

1   He defines quality of life in terms of happiness, but does not then discuss the meaning of happiness beyond saying that it is contingent upon the satisfaction of a range of wants. Other researchers have considered the nature of happiness in more depth. Historically, the meaning ascribed to the term has varied, from an internal psychological state akin to euphoria, to wellbeing. This debate will be explored more fully below when we look at subjective approaches to quality of life.

2   The approach is at odds with those who relate quality of life not to wants, but to needs, as does McCall (1980). He argues that 'wants' are a poor basis for defining quality of life because they vary so widely between individuals, whereas 'needs', he believes, are universal, and can be defined with reference to the work of Maslow (Maslow 1954). Maslow proposed that human needs can be arranged in a hierarchy. At the base of the hierarchy are fundamental physiological needs, such as that for food and water. When these are satisfied, the human being seeks to fulfil his or her needs for safety and·security, and the satisfaction of these needs is followed in turn by the need to belong, the need to be held in esteem, and the need to 'self-actualise', or develop one's potential. McCall then goes on to develop an approach to quality of life based on an assessment of the extent to which an individual has the resources necessary to meet these needs.

3   Liu's decision to leave out the 'spiritual' or subjective components means that his approach to measuring quality of life amounts to little more than an assessment of material circumstances (Huxley 1986). This leads him into difficulty, because it

was discovered many years ago that there is only a tenuous link between objective indicators of quality of life and people's evaluation of their own life satisfaction. For instance, Rescher (1972) noted that although the material circumstances of Americans, as measured by indicators such as life expectancy, income, and social welfare expenditure had increased, their level of happiness had declined; and Campbell *et al.* (1976) noted that the American nation, which had been known and criticised for its materialistic values, was now asking itself whether in fact the good life could be measured in terms of consumer goods. Furthermore, a number of studies conducted in the mid-seventies empirically demonstrated that the objective conditions of life are only marginally related to the subjective experience of a better quality of life (Campbell *et al.* 1976, Schneider 1975).

That 'objective' measurements of a person's circumstances often differ from 'subjective' evaluations of her or his life satisfaction is one of the most interesting findings of the social indicators movement. This so-called 'satisfaction paradox' takes the two basic forms shown in Box 2.2.

**Box 2.2 The satisfaction paradox**

- people who live in rather privileged circumstances while expressing dissatisfaction about their quality of life – Zapf (1984) has referred to such people as the 'frustrated privileged';
- people who express satisfaction with the quality of their lives even though an 'objective' appraisal of their circumstances would identify these as unsatisfactory.

There may be a number of explanations for the latter phenomenon. People's evaluations of their quality of life may result not from comparisons with the whole of the society of which they are a part, but only from comparisons with local reference groups. Kozma and Stones (1988) argued that people tend to say that they

are satisfied with their life circumstances because they believe that
to be the socially desirable response to make. It is also possible that
people in poverty may simply resign themselves to their lot and
therefore adapt their standards to the poor situation in which they
find themselves.

More recent work on the paradox has been undertaken by Olson
and Schober (1993), who draw upon two psychological theories:
Seligman's theory of learned helplessness (Seligman 1979) and
Festinger's theory of the minimisation of cognitive dissonance
(Festinger 1957). Seligman's theory explains the behaviour of individuals who learn that the probability of changing an undesirable
situation is the same irrespective of any actions they may take.
Festinger's theory asserts that people try to be consistent in their
behaviours and their beliefs, so that if individuals find themselves in
circumstances in which their behaviours and beliefs are incongruent
or out of phase, they will act in various ways in order to relieve the
tension caused. Olson and Schober suggest that the experiences of
people in poverty may lead them to believe that they are unable, by
their own efforts, to influence their circumstances for the better.
Having learned that they are helpless, they will then adjust to their
situation by rationalising the cognitive dissonance arising from the
stigma of poverty and avowing that they are satisfied with their
material circumstances.

The difficulties with objective social indicators discussed above
led some researchers to be dissatisfied with the objective approach
to quality of life and to focus instead on the development of subjective approaches to its measurement. Aspects of their work are
discussed in the next section.

## Subjective social indicators

All subjective indicators of quality of life make the two assumptions shown in Box 2.3.

Subjective social indicators offer a range of techniques through
which such self-assessments can be made. Andrews (1974) was an
early worker in this field, and has offered these four reasons for
developing subjective indicators of quality of life:

**Box 2.3** Key assumptions of subjective indicators

● The concept of quality of life refers to a person's degree of satisfaction with certain aspects of his or her life.
● The individual concerned is in the best position to judge the amount of satisfaction she or he feels.

1  They provide direct measures of individuals' evaluations of their own well-being.
2  They enable the relationships between life concerns to be explored.
3  They provide a check on the adequacy of a range of a set of objective measures.
4  They lead to knowledge which is useful in designing pro- grammes whose aim is the enhancement of individual well-being.

Research in the subjective indicator field has its roots in the work of Cantril (1965), who interviewed a cross-section of people from var- ious countries to determine what aspects of life they considered important from positive and negative points of view, and where they scaled their personal standing in the present and the future. One of the largest studies of this type was conducted by Andrews and Withey (1976), whose research involved interviews with over 5,000 Americans and provided base-line data on the distribution of perceptions of well-being across US society. The basic concepts in their model concerned well-being at several levels of specificity. At the most general level were global indicators referring to life as a whole; the next level addressed concerns, consisting of aspects of life about which people have feelings. These were divided into domains (such as job, family life and neighbourhood) which could be evaluated in terms of criteria (such as privacy, comfort and security). Similar work was conducted in the UK by Abrams (1976). Abrams invited respondents to give an overall assessment of their life situation in terms of twelve domains, including housing, health, neighbourhood, job, family life and financial situation.

One of the most striking features of this part of the literature is the lack of consensus on the nature and definition of the underlying construct 'well-being'. Terms such as 'satisfaction', 'morale' and 'happiness' are often used interchangeably (Zautra and Hempel 1982). Following Peschar (1977), this discussion will first evaluate the idea that self-reports of happiness give a useful index of quality of life, and then focus on the measurement of well-being.

Happiness is a major goal in contemporary Western society. Most people would probably agree that it is better to enjoy life than to suffer, and would endorse policies whose aim is to create greater happiness for greater numbers of people (Veenhoven 1995). The belief that people can become happier in the right circumstances is rooted in a humanistic view of people as autonomous beings who are able to improve their conditions by the use of reason; a view which Veenhoven (1994) considers forms the ideological basis of welfare states. The view that we ought to strive to improve happiness is also grounded in the enlightenment tradition, although the preference of happiness over unhappiness was prefigured in ancient Greek moral philosophy: Aristotle asserted that happiness is the only value which is final and sufficient. It is final because all else is merely a means of achieving it; and sufficient because, once happiness is attained, nothing else is desired (Diener 1993). In the nineteenth century, this view formed the basis of the utilitarian doctrine of trying to achieve 'the greatest happiness for the greatest number'.

Inevitably, there is disagreement in the literature about the nature of happiness and about its relationship to quality of life. The historical development of the concept is discussed by Tatarkiewicz (1976), who explains that in early times, 'happiness' was simply another word for 'success'. Then, throughout antiquity and the Middle Ages, it signified the state of a perfect human being who possessed the highest virtues and goods. Modern times have tended to reduce happiness to pleasure. Tatarkiewicz suggests that the evolution of the concept has tended to swing between these two extremes: happiness as perfection and as pleasure.

The modern literature continues to reflect these approaches. Malcolm-Gill (1984), for instance, reduces happiness to an internal psychological state akin to pleasure or euphoria, while Bradburn and Noll (1969) relate it to well-being, a much broader concept in the tradition of Aristotle's 'eudaemonia' (human flourishing).

One of the problems in using self-reports of happiness as indices of quality of life is that happiness appears to be a consequence of the gap between expectation and achievement (Shin and Johnson 1978, Mason and Faulkenberry 1978). So conditions that are objectively identical can elicit very different responses from different individuals, while subjectively similar responses can result from widely differing objective situations (Callebaut 1980). As Kennedy *et al.* (1978) comment, different individuals can be satisfied or dissatisfied with the same objective conditions. Many nurses will have seen examples of this paradox in their own clinical practice. For instance, it is not unusual to find older people who strongly resist the opportunity to take a place in a residential home that has good medical and social facilities, three hot meals a day, and plenty of companionship, preferring instead to live on their own in conditions that any 'objective' appraisal would find squalid and unsatisfactory.

McCall (1980) suggests that human needs are specific and limited, whereas wants are potentially boundless. He argues that the satisfaction of human needs is a necessary but not sufficient condition for happiness and satisfaction. A person will be satisfied or unsatisfied to the extent to which basic needs and major wants are filled. It is because wants vary from individual to individual that the correlation between objective conditions, and the subjective evaluation of those conditions, is relatively weak.

Seashore (1974) offers another explanation. He refers to human adaptability, arguing that being satisfied is a common coping response which offers a means of defining one's situation in an acceptable light and thereby coming to terms with it. These two mechanisms may, of course, operate simultaneously. Although Veenhoven (1991) rejects the assumptions on which this paradox is based, many other authors consider that it throws into doubt the validity and usefulness of self-reports of happiness as an index of quality of life (Shin and Johnson 1978, Mason and Faulkenberry 1978, Callebaut 1980).

The discussion now turns to the subjective assessment of well-being. Diener (1984) suggests that subjective well-being has these three characteristics:

1  It is subjective, in that it resides within the experience of the individual.
2  It is not simply the absence of negative factors but also has a positive component.
3  It is based on a global assessment of life rather than a narrow evaluation of one or a few life domains.

Veenhoven (1994) defines well-being as the degree to which a person judges the overall quality of his or her life as a whole in a favourable light. He asserts that individuals' evaluations of their life satisfaction are influenced by two components: affects and thoughts. The affective component is the hedonic level, comprising the pleasantness experienced in moods, emotions and feelings. Campbell *et al.* (1976) define the cognitive component as the perceived discrepancy between aspiration and achievement, suggesting that it ranges from the perception of fulfilment to that of deprivation. They argue that satisfaction implies a judgemental or cognitive experience while happiness suggests an experience of feeling or affect.

Researchers have found life satisfaction to be strongly influenced by health (Larson 1978, Zautra and Hempel 1984, Lehman 1993) and various other factors including one's degree of social interaction (Najman and Levine 1981). Carley (1981) suggests that while few things may be simpler than dreaming up evaluation scales and then finding a few hundred obliging people to tick the boxes, it is not easy to interpret or judge the significance of their responses. This is partly because, as we have seen, people may respond differently to the same set of circumstances. Campbell *et al.* (1976) have also noted a 'happiness barrier', or a tendency for people to respond in an overly positive manner at a global level while being critical of their life situation at the level of specific issues. A related problem concerns the difficulty of separating out the effects of demographic and other variables on subjective responses. For instance, Huxley (1986) reports that young people return high scores on happiness but low scores on life satisfaction, while older people score more highly on life satisfaction and have lower scores on happiness.

The final issue related to subjective social indicators concerns their relevance for policy. Although Andrews (1974) argues that subjective social indicators would be useful in policy planning, Carley (1981) considers that global measures of quality of life remain vague and general, and finds it difficult to imagine their value to policy is beyond that of the average Gallup poll.

## Summary

In this chapter, we have examined some of the literature produced by workers in the field of social indicators research. This represents the earliest systematic discussion of quality of life, and contains a number of important themes and debates, including the following:

- Is quality of life best regarded as an objective phenomenon that can be measured without reference to the individuals in question?
- Is it essentially an internal, subjective state related to happiness or well-being?

The subjective–objective debate is an issue about which nurses may have strong opinions. Sutcliffe and Holmes (1991), who probably express the views of many nurses, suggest that no one can or should make judgements about the quality of life of another person. In so far as they are opposing the kind of overbearing paternalism which enables one person to feel competent as a judge of the private sensations and emotions of another, such as pain, nausea or perhaps degree of happiness, then this position seems reasonable. In the light of research which shows a discrepancy between patients' and doctors' ratings of the outcome of therapy, it seems even more reasonable (Orth-Gomer *et al.* 1979, Thomas and Lyttle 1980, Jachuk and Brierly 1982). However, this argument assumes that pain, nausea or the degree of happiness can be taken as markers of quality of life without demonstrating that this is so; and it also assumes the sufficiency of these internal phenomena: that they and they alone determine quality of life. But it can be argued that quality of life is at least partially constituted by elements which are shared with others: aspects of the physical environment, perhaps, or the quality of one's interpersonal relationships. If this is the case, then it is difficult to sustain the view that quality of life is an entirely private affair.

# Chapter 3
# The quality adjusted life year (QALY)

In the previous chapter, we saw that quality of life is commonly regarded as a measurable characteristic of individuals or groups of people. We found that the earliest systematic attempts to measure it were made by social indicators researchers, and we noted several important characteristics of their work. These included the debate between those who regard quality of life as an objective state that can be measured by collecting social statistics of various kinds; and those who define it in subjective terms, arguing that the level of quality of life is something that can only be judged by each individual concerned. We also noted that a considerable discrepancy often exists between subjective and objective measures of quality of life, and a number of explanations for this were discussed.

Of course, interest in the concept of quality of life is not restricted to social indicators researchers. The concept is also used by people who work in a broad range of practical professions, including politicians, social workers, teachers, nurses and many others. In fact, anyone whose work involves promoting the well-being of other people could probably claim an interest in quality of life – as could those individuals whose lives are affected by their work.

In this chapter and the next, we shall consider ways in which the concept is put to use by medical practitioners. The growth in interest in quality of life in medicine has been phenomenal. *Index Medicus*, the index of medical literature, first introduced quality of life as a category in 1966. In that year, only one quality of life article was published. Between 1981 and 1986, 1,902 articles were published, while between 1991 and 1996 the number rose to 8,820. This chapter critically examines papers from that body of literature which introduce the idea of the 'quality adjusted life year', or QALY.

Many Western governments are concerned with the increasing cost of health and social care and are keen to find ways of reducing or at least limiting the growth in costs while maintaining an adequate health service. A specific example of the problem, and an attempt to resolve it, can be found in the United States. The state of Oregon was so concerned with the growth of its Medicaid budget (which funds health care for those who are unable to afford private health insurance) that it undertook an extensive priority setting exercise, in which members of the public were asked to rank various treatments in order of their importance, with a view to not providing services that were ranked below a certain point.

It is often argued that although the financial resources available to pay for health services are limited, the demand for those services is potentially infinite. If this premise is accepted, then it becomes necessary to choose which health services to buy and to decide how much money to spend on each of them, as Gudex (1986) suggests.

In the commercial world, decisions about the range of services that ought to be provided for a particular need are often resolved in the market place. For instance, people are free to shop for their weekly groceries at any one of a range of supermarkets or local shops, and they can buy whatever they like within the limits of their budget. Supermarkets that do not provide what the customer wants will eventually go out of business.

The influence of market forces of this kind on British health care was effectively suspended when the National Health Service was created (Culyer 1984), and until recently, funding decisions were either taken centrally or delegated to a complex bureaucratic structure of regional and local health authorities. For many years, the only formal mechanism for resource allocation with statutory power was RAWP, the formula of the Resource Allocation Working Party, which was created as a means of diverting money from London to the regions (Carr-Hill 1991). It has been argued that strategies for funding at the local level often lacked coherence and were unduly influenced by local medical politics; and accusations of 'allocation by shroud-waving' (money goes to the medical speciality that can produce the most horror stories) or 'allocation by decibel' (money goes to the consultant who can shout the loudest) were often made (Crisp 1989).

This situation has been changed to some extent by recent health reforms. Under the new system, various Trusts compete with one another to win contracts to provide medical services for purchasing authorities and fund-holding GP practices. However, the new system does not resolve the resource allocation problem but simply displaces it, making local health service managers responsible for what was once a problem for central government.

For Lockwood (1988), a natural response to the problem of how to allocate limited resources is simply to say that one should spend one's money where it will do the most good. He notes that this raises two questions:

1  What do we mean by the most good?
2  How can we discriminate between alternative programmes in terms of the good which they achieve?

One kind of good that health care may achieve is saving lives. An appropriate measure of this is the overall extension of life expectancy generated by a particular therapy, expressed as years of life gained. Some years ago, Gould (1975) strongly advocated this approach, arguing that we should give a very high priority to the aim of maximising aggregate years of life gained. He recognised that this policy would divert a large part of the health budget to preventing accidents and suicide, while a smaller but still substantial amount would go to preventing and curing heart and lung disease. Much less would be spent on cancer, which is predominantly a disease of the latter half of life, and which therefore contributes relatively little to the sum total of life years lost. Gould also advocated that no money should be made available for the treatment of old people with serious illnesses.

Gould assumes that the primary goal of health care is to extend the length of life, and if this were so then years of life gained would constitute a fair criterion of success. However, this basic assumption can be challenged. Obvious examples of the enormous range of current health services that are not significantly life-extending are routine dental surgery, treatments for unpleasant conditions such as arthritis, and probably the greater part of nursing care. Later in this chapter, we will also see that many medical practitioners justify their therapies not by their life-extending properties, but because they have an impact on quality of life. In summary, analyses that focus exclusively on life years gained are of limited value. For this reason, health economists have attempted to develop measures of outcome which balance the life extending and the life enhancing aspects of care: 'quality and quantity of life have somehow to be rendered mutually commensurable' (Lockwood 1988:35).

The second problem faced by health economists is knowing how to discriminate between various programmes in terms of the 'good' which they offer. In many cases, clinical research tells us what outcomes to expect from the introduction of a new therapy, test or health care programme, and data on the financial cost of such programmes are readily available. However, it is difficult to compare different interventions in terms of their cost-effectiveness. According to Yin *et al.* (1995), the problem is caused by our inability to measure the value of health states; if it were possible to measure this, then it would also be possible to compare various therapies for different clinical conditions and to rank them in terms of (1) cost and (2) their impact on health.

The technical name for comparing the costs of different procedures with common units of outcome, or 'utility based units', is 'cost-utility analysis', and the most commonly used utility based unit is probably the 'quality adjusted life year', or QALY.

The QALY is an attempt to provide a basis for resource allocation decisions which values both quantitative and qualitative outcomes. In Britain, it has been advocated by Alan Williams of the Centre for Health Economics at the University of York, and the approach is fully described in discussion papers produced by that centre (Gudex 1986, Gudex and Kind 1989). Williams describes the QALY in the following way:

> [We] need a simple, versatile, measure of success which incorporates both life expectancy and quality of life, and which reflects the values and ethics of the community served. The . . . QALY . . . measure fulfils such a role. The essence of a QALY is that it takes one year of healthy life expectancy to be worth 1, but regards a year of unhealthy life expectancy as worth less than 1. Its precise value is lower the worse the

quality of life of the unhealthy person (which is what the 'quality adjusted' bit is all about). If being dead is worth zero, it is, in principle, possible for a QALY to be negative, i.e. for the quality of someone's life to be judged as worse than being dead. The general idea is that a beneficial health care activity is one that generates a positive amount of QALYs, and an efficient health care activity is one where the cost-per-QALY is as low as it can be.

(Williams 1985:3)

Crisp (1989) offers a hypothetical example of the QALY at work, shown in Box 3.1.

---

**Box 3.1  Example of the QALY at work**

Crisp describes the case of a patient who is expected to live in perfect health for ten years after having a heart transplant. In such a case, the gain in QALYs is 10 × 1 = 10. In another hypothetical case, a patient undergoing treatment for leukaemia may also live for ten years, but with a quality of life which is diminished by the illness. If it is assumed that her quality of life is only half as good as it would be if she were in full health, then the QALYs produced by treating her work out at 10 × 0.5 = 5. It is now possible to work out costs-per-QALY. If heart transplant costs £100,000, the cost-per-QALY is £100,000/10 = £10,000; whereas the cost-per-QALY for a course of chemotherapy costing £20,000 is £20,000/5 = £4,000. In this case, treating leukaemia would be deemed a more efficient use of resources than transplanting hearts.

---

A great many examples in the literature of research have followed a similar procedure. For instance:

● McIntyre *et al.* (1994) conducted a cost-utility analysis of various strategies for immunising children against influenza;

- Kamlet *et al.* (1995) evaluated three maintenance treatments for chronic depression;
- Geelhoed *et al.* (1994) conducted cost-utility analysis of hormone replacement therapy as opposed to lifestyle interventions for hip fracture.

The QALY has had an impact on health policy and the management of health services in the UK (Gudex 1986), in the US (Haddorn 1991) and elsewhere. It has also been the focus of vigorous critical debate between health economists, ethical philosophers and health professionals. Internal criticisms concern the technical procedures used to generate QALYs and the assumptions upon which these procedures rest. External criticisms concern the broader social and economic context in which QALYs are used, the purposes to which they are put, and the possible consequences of their use. These two groups of criticisms are discussed in more detail below.

## Internal criticisms of the QALY

Internal criticisms of the QALY focus on the mechanism used to attach values to various health states, and the validity and usefulness of these evaluations. Utility measures such as the QALY enable people to express their preference for various health states. The literature describes several different ways of obtaining these preferences. One is to classify patients into categories based on their responses to questions about their functional status, as for instance the European Quality of Life Measure (EUROQOL). Another is to ask patients to assign a single rating to their overall health by such means as a rating scale or techniques like the standard gamble, time trade-off, or willingness to pay (Bakker and van der Linden 1995).

Williams (1985), who is the architect of the QALY in Great Britain, used the Rosser Classification of Illness States, which combines various categories of distress and disability, as a basis for evaluating various health states (see Table 3.1). Seventy respondents were asked to classify various combinations of disability and distress according to their undesirability, using a score where

*Table 3.1.* Rosser's Classification of Illness States

---

Levels of disability

---

I     No disability

II    Slight social disability

III   Severe social disability and/or slight impairment of performance
      at work
      Able to do all housework except very heavy tasks

IV    Choice of work or performance at work very severely limited
      Housewives and old people able to do light housework only but
      able to go out shopping.

V     Unable to undertake any paid employment
      Unable to continue any education
      Old people confined to home except for escorted outings and
      short walks, and unable to do shopping
      Housewives able to perform only a few simple tasks

VI    Confined to chair or to wheelchair or able to move around in the
      house only with support from an assistant

VII   Confined to bed

VIII  Unconscious

---

Levels of distress: A = No distress; B = Mild distress;
C = Moderate distress; D = Severe distress.

1 = healthy and 0 = dead. The resulting scores are reproduced as
Rosser's Valuation Matrix (see Table 3.2). The mean score for each
combination of disability and distress is represented by the figure
in the cell.

*Table 3.2.* Rosser's Valuation Matrix

| Disability | | | Distress | |
|---|---|---|---|---|
| | A | B | C | D |
| I | 1.000 | 0.995 | 0.990 | 0.967 |
| II | 0.990 | 0.986 | 0.973 | 0.932 |
| III | 0.980 | 0.972 | 0.956 | 0.912 |
| IV | 0.964 | 0.956 | 0.942 | 0.870 |
| V | 0.946 | 0.935 | 0.900 | 0.700 |
| VI | 0.875 | 0.845 | 0.680 | 0.000 |
| VII | 0.677 | 0.564 | 0.000 | −1.486 |
| VIII | −1.028 | n.a. | n.a. | n.a. |

Fixed points: 1 = Healthy; 0 = Dead.
n.a. = Not applicable.

The Rosser Valuation Matrix, which lies at the heart of the QALY procedure, can be criticised for the assumptions it embodies. The first is that of correspondence.

## *The assumption of correspondence*

This is the assumption that the scores generated by the Rosser procedure will correspond with people's everyday evaluations of various degrees of health or ill-health. This assumption has two parts:

1 that when people are asked to make hypothetical decisions about resource allocation they will employ quality of life as a criterion;
2 that they will define quality of life in terms of disability and distress.

These are examined below.

## Part 1

In a recent empirical study from Norway, Nord (1993) asked subjects how they felt a hospital should prioritise between two patients admitted within a few hours of each other. Both were described as being in a life-threatening condition. It was said that one could regain full health if treated, and the other could be given a life of moderate pain and dependency on crutches for walking. The hospital might not manage to operate on both in time. In the subject's opinion, how ought the hospital to prioritise between the two?

Forty-eight of the subjects in Nord's study (79 per cent) felt that the two patients should be treated in the order in which they were admitted to the hospital. Only nine subjects (15 per cent) were in favour of giving priority to the patient with the better expected outcome. Thirty-one subjects in the majority group of forty-eight explicitly argued in terms of equality in value of life and/or entitlement to treatment.

Nord accepts that the sample used is too small to support broad generalisations, but argues that health economists should determine people's ethical preferences in matters of prioritising, rather than taking it for granted that their own values are shared by the general public.

In a second and more recent study, Nord *et al.* (1995) conducted a two-stage survey in which a cross-section of Australians were questioned about the importance of costs in setting priorities in health care. Generally, respondents felt it unfair to discriminate against patients with a high-cost illness and argued that costs should not be a major factor in prioritising. The majority maintained this view even when confronted with the implication that the total number of people who could be treated would be reduced, and their own chances of receiving treatment if they fell ill was smaller. Nord concludes that the economist's concern with efficiency of allocation is not shared by the general public, who may see the cost-effectiveness approach to assigning priorities in health care as imposing an excessively simple value system on resource allocation decision making.

**Part 2**

The second part of the assumption of correspondence is that quality of life can be expressed as a function of disability and distress. Although Williams accepts that this definition is crude and needs refinement (Williams 1985), he defends its use on the grounds that physical mobility and freedom from distress are fundamental aspects of the life experience, and that without them, we cannot perform the activities of daily living and engage in normal social interaction. This may be true, but for Rawles (1989) it is not the point. He argues that to equate the value of human life with the absence of disability and distress is to undervalue human existence very greatly. He claims that life is valued for infinitely more reasons than the absence of suffering.

The assumption is also challenged by Loomes and McKenzie (1989), who note the rather stringent conditions that Williams imposed on his respondents. They were instructed to:

- think of each health state as existing for the same length of time;
- judge each state on the basis of its intrinsic 'enjoyability';
- evaluate all states as if the respondent were 'in them now';
- be uninfluenced by the likely prognosis of the sufferer (Williams 1981).

Loomes and McKenzie argue that the value attached to a health state ought not to be considered independent either of the time spent in it, or of the health states preceding or expected to follow it. For example, the grading of a particular combination of disability and distress may well differ if experienced for a long or short time; and an acute, self-limiting illness will have a different meaning from one whose expected outcome is death. Loomes and McKenzie also argue that people's evaluation of health states will vary with their attitude to risk, which should therefore be held constant when comparisons are made between subjects.

In recent work by Kiebert *et al.* (1994), 199 patients with cancer were asked to indicate the importance of the following: age at the time of decision, having a partner, having children, inability to work due to side-effects of treatment, the nature of the side-effects, disease-related life expectancy, and base-line quality of life. The results indicated that six of the seven factors listed were of considerable to great importance when a treatment choice had to be made. The negative effect of treatment on the ability to work did not seem to be a very important consideration. This study is significant because it shows people's evaluation of various states of health and illness is influenced by personal circumstances of the kind that were held constant in Williams's work.

## The assumption of stability

This is the assumption that people have a set of internal preferences or evaluations which is relatively stable, and that these are accurately represented by the numbers they assign to various health states. However, Mulkay *et al.* (1987) argue that the values given by respondents must be seen in the context of the highly structured and artificial social situation produced by the researcher: a context in which the respondents answer a very specific question in a predetermined format. Mulkay *et al.* can find no reason to suppose that the responses given in these circumstances will represent responses to situations in real life.

## The assumption of quantification

This assumption is fundamental to the procedure for constructing QALYs. It concerns the requirement for respondents to make precise numerical assessments of situations described by the analyst. The method of analysis assumes that the numbers respondents assign have some real meaning for them in ordinary situations, and that these numbers express quantifications already implicit in individual respondents' scales of preference. Carr-Hill (1991) rejects this assumption, arguing that index numbers are not neutral observations but the product of a highly specific set of technical procedures, and that they serve the interests of particular groups. He is suspicious of factor analyses in which responses to a series of questions are combined in elaborate exercises with dubious statistical validity and then given pretentious labels. He suggests that such techniques may be particularly tempting to researchers dealing with responses to questions of little interest and concern to the people being interviewed.

Haddorn's criticism of this assumption questions the meaning of the numbers generated by the QALY procedure. He asks what it means to speak of someone having a one-tenth-normal quality of life, and doubts that it is possible to quantify something as amorphous and ill defined as the quality of life (Haddorn 1991). He also believes that some of the results gained when the QALY was used as part of the Oregon priority setting exercise are quite at odds with common sense. On one occasion, for example, respondents awarded the same numerical values to an upset stomach and to burns over large areas of the body.

## External criticisms of the QALY

External criticisms of the QALY focus on:

- the economic and political environment in which the system is used;
- the purposes to which it is put;
- the potential consequences of its use.

The QALY was developed in response to the political argument that demand for health care is potentially infinite, while the financial resources available to meet that demand are strictly limited. Rawles (1989) and Rawles and Rawles (1990) argue that infinite demand is no more true for the National Health Service than it is for a free public lavatory. Rawles (1989) says that at each stage of life, from birth to death, the incidence of disease, the nature and cost of its treatment, the requirements for preventive measures, and the loss of life from various causes are all known with a high degree of precision. Harris (1987) argues that the limits on health care expenditure are much more stringent than they need or ought to be, and suggests that health has a stronger moral claim upon the nation's financial resources than does, for example, defence. Rawles (1989) argues that additional funding of 2.0 per cent per year would enable the National Health Service to keep pace with demographic, technological and policy changes. While acknowledging that this is a substantial increase, Rawles claims that it is 'a long way short of infinity' (Rawles 1989:144).

Harris argues that the QALY is logically defective. He suggests that its plausibility depends on our accepting the generalisation that, given the choice, a person would prefer a shorter, healthier life to a longer period of survival in a state of discomfort. Harris argues that, although this assumption enables one to claim that the best treatment for an individual is the one that supplies the most QALYs, it does not follow that treatments yielding more QALYs are preferable to those yielding fewer where different people are involved. For example, where the choice is between three years of discomfort for me or my immediate death on the one hand, and one year of health for you, or your immediate death on the other, I am not necessarily committed to the judgement that you ought to be saved rather than me (Harris 1988).

Harris's criticism of the QALY rests on the belief that the value of one life cannot be traded off against the value of another. He states that the value of someone's life is, primarily and overwhelmingly, its value to him or her; and that the wrong done when an individual's life is cut short is a wrong to that individual (Harris 1987).

Harris (1987, 1988) also objects to the QALY because he believes that it will bias the distribution of health care resources away from some groups in society, while placing others at a relative advantage. He argues, for instance, that elderly people will be disadvantaged because money spent on their health care will not generate as many QALYs as money spent on younger people. Donaldson *et al.* (1988) suggest that the QALY will be less sensitive to changes in the health status of elderly people than will programme-specific measures such as the Crichton Royal Behavioural Rating Scale.

Singer *et al.* (1995) discuss the impact that QALY thinking has on people with disability. Their quality of life is ranked on the QALY scale below that of those without disability or illness. It follows that, all other things being equal, we can gain more QALYs by saving the lives of those without disability or illness than by saving the lives of those who are disadvantaged in these ways. It is sometimes argued that this puts the disadvantaged people under a form of double jeopardy: they not only suffer from the disability or illness, but because of it a low priority is given to health care that can preserve their lives, and this is unfair.

Lockwood (1988) takes issue with Harris's argument that the QALY is unjust to older people. Although he does not deny that it is to their disadvantage, he argues that, all else being equal, it is preferable to give a scarce resource to a younger person rather than an older one because the older one has had a 'fair innings'. Lockwood argues that the real problem with the QALY is that it is not sensitive to situational factors such as the number of a person's dependents. He believes the key question to be: does the death or continued ill-health of the patient compromise the capacity of the dependents to flourish as human beings? If the answer is yes, he suggests that the needs of the dependents should also be taken into account.

Finally, the QALY is criticised for using the concept of quality of life in a manner radically different from the historical one. Aiken (1982) shows that within the liberal tradition, 'quality of life' has described the material and social goods which persons must have if they are to achieve that minimal level of well-being which enables them to live as moral entities, and thus to pursue the 'good life'. This liberal tradition has its roots in the work of nineteenth-century reformers who stressed the need for basic material amenities to satisfy physical needs. They believed that all humans are entitled to liberty, a minimal level of physical well-being, and the institutions to guarantee this. The social indicators movement continues this tradition, because its declared purpose is to promote quality of life. Aiken (1982) contrasts this egalitarian use of the concept with an exclusionary use that he associates with the QALY. The traditional prescriptive uses of 'quality of life' promote this value; but the 'exclusionary' use cites 'quality of life' as providing a criterion for excluding some people from the moral community, and concomitantly from normal standards of moral treatment. Because a person's quality of life is below the desirable level, that person's life is judged to be not worth living, and we are justified in treating them accordingly. The QALY uses quality of life as a criterion for including or excluding individuals and groups from access to health care resources. It is therefore exclusionary in Aiken's sense.

## Summary

In this chapter, we have discussed one way in which the concept of quality of life is employed in the medical field – the quality adjusted life year, or QALY.

The idea of the QALY arose in the context of a particular economic and political situation. The argument went that the potential demand for the health services is infinite while the resources available to meet it are strictly limited. Health economists created the QALY as a means of balancing the life-extending and the life-enhancing aspects of care. It purports to offer a single unit of measurement which can be used to calculate the value of various therapies in a way which, while not being strictly scientific, is at least more objective than any other approach available at the moment. It also appears to have the benefit of reflecting underlying social preferences.

Philosophers, health economists and others have offered a number of criticisms of the QALY, and some of these have been reviewed above. For the moment, particular attention is drawn to the criticisms shown in Box 3.2.

---

**Box 3.2 Key criticisms of the QALY**

- People are asked to attach numbers to various combinations of disability and distress, using a range of techniques.
- Carr-Hill (1991) observes that index numbers are not neutral observations upon the world, but the product of a highly specific set of technical procedures and serve the interests of particular groups.

---

As Paton (1995) observes, a great many groups in society have a stake in the outcome of resource allocation decisions, and not all will be satisfied by the outcomes of QALY calculations.

These facts tend to weaken any suggestion that the QALY is objective in any scientific sense. It is interesting to note that a number of the issues in the earlier discussion of social indicators research are also present here. We find once again that quality of life research does not take place in a political vacuum. As social indicators research emerged from a political concern with certain social and economic phenomena, and social indicators themselves were designed to be of use in formulating policy, so QALY research exists against a background of concern about the rising costs of health service care and a preoccupation with effectiveness and efficiency. This context is important, because it defines a set of assumptions which in turn guide the questions that researchers consider worth answering and the research methods that they use.

The next chapter examines a third field of quality of life research, focusing on the use of quality of life as an outcome measure in research designed to evaluate the effectiveness of various medical therapies.

# Chapter 4
# Quality of life and medical research

In recent years, medical researchers have shown increasing interest in the concept of quality of life. The rate of growth in the literature is illustrated by entering 'quality of life' as a search term in Medline (the computerised index to medical literature), which shows that there were no published papers on quality of life in the medical literature before 1966. In that year, Elkington published a paper entitled 'Medicine and the quality of life' (Elkington 1966). In the four years following the publication of Elkington's paper, eight further papers were published on the topic. Since 1970, growth of interest in the field has been exponential (Table 4.1).

*Table 4.1* Number of references to 'quality of life' in Medline, 1966–96

| From | To | Total number of papers published | Total number of clinical trials published | Clinical trials as percentage of whole |
|------|------|------|------|------|
| 1966 | 1970 | 9 | 0 | 0 |
| 1971 | 1975 | 182 | 2 | 1.10 |
| 1976 | 1980 | 1,165 | 25 | 2.15 |
| 1981 | 1985 | 1,902 | 77 | 4.05 |
| 1986 | 1990 | 4,606 | 337 | 7.30 |
| 1991 | 1996 | 8,820 | 900 | 10.20 |

The medical literature examines a number of issues. It contains philosophical papers which discuss the meaning of quality of life, methodological papers which discuss its subjective or objective nature and describe ways in which quality of life can be measured, papers which discuss the relationship of quality of life to health status (for a review see Bowling 1991), and yet other papers which, as we saw in Chapter 3, bring quality of life to bear on the resource allocation debate.

A number of reasons have been suggested for the growth of interest in the quality of life in the medical literature. Hayry (1991) suggests that, in addition to their role in the allocation of scarce medical resources, quality of life measurements also facilitate clinical decision making and assist patients to make autonomous decisions. He considers that a physician who knows the expected values of alternative treatments, in terms of the quantity and quality of life, is in a good position to make considered choices for his or her patients; and suggests that patients themselves should be fully involved in these decisions.

The conventional justification for measuring quality of life in medicine is that it provides information which usefully complements data on the life-preserving properties of medical interventions. This argument was propounded by Najman and Levine (1981), who suggested that if technologically based medical care were to be judged on the purely quantitative criteria of increasing longevity, then only a small fraction of the care delivered would meet the required standard. These authors suggested that most medical care is not, in fact, intended to increase the length of life, but is provided in order to relieve symptoms, improve mental health, restore functioning, or reduce pain and discomfort, and they argued that health care ought to be evaluated in terms of the impact that it has on quality of life. The activities and procedures that produce the largest improvement should receive the most support.

In view of this argument, it is interesting to observe that only a relatively small percentage of published quality of life papers are described in Medline as 'clinical trials', and therefore examine the impact of a medical intervention upon the quality of patients' lives (see Table 4.1). From 1966 to 1996, a little over 8 per cent of all published medical quality of life literature described clinical trials. Table 4.1 also shows that, if the number of clinical trials is examined in blocks of five years, clinical trials have only recently made up 10 per cent of all quality of life papers published.

It is beyond the limitations of this book to examine every part of the medical literature on quality of life. As it has been claimed that the importance of medical interventions is related to their impact upon the quality of patients' lives, we shall focus on and evaluate the literature which uses quality of life as an outcome measure in clinical trials.

Medline was used to identify a series of quality of life outcome studies published in the medical literature over a six-month period in 1995. Review articles were excluded. The following analysis of that literature is concerned with the four issues shown in Box 4.1.

---

**Box 4.1 Key issues in analysing outcome studies**

- the extent to which quality of life criteria are used to assess the benefits of health care;
- the nature of quality of life indicators used;
- the adequacy of research designs;
- the findings of the studies evaluated.

---

This approach is adapted from Najman and Levine (1981), and has also been used by Draper (1994).

Table 4.2 confirms that quality of life has become a popular outcome measure in medical research, with studies published in a number of different medical specialities. The procedures discussed include medical and surgical treatments for gastric disease (mentioned three times), treatment for intermittent claudication (mentioned once), surgical treatment of heart disease (mentioned three times), medical treatment of heart disease (mentioned once), rehousing of people with a learning disability (mentioned once), surgical treatments for laryngeal cancer, prostate cancer and eye

*Table 4.2* Research questions addressed by a series of fourteen outcome studies

| Number | Authors | Question addressed |
| --- | --- | --- |
| 1 | Buhl *et al.* (1995) | Comparison of effect of two methods of reconstruction following gastrectomy on quality of life |
| 2 | Currie *et al.* (1995) | Assessment of the impact of various forms of treatment for claudication on quality of life |
| 3 | Dagnan *et al.* (1995) | What is the effect on quality of life of moving people with learning disabilities from hospital to community homes? |
| 4 | De Santo *et al.* (1995) | What impact does surgical treatment of cancer of the larynx have on quality of life? |
| 5 | Freitas *et al.* (1995) | What is the impact of photorefractive keratectomy on visual functioning and quality of life? |
| 6 | Kumar *et al.* (1995) | What is the quality of life of octogenarians following heart surgery? |
| 7 | Lim *et al.* (1995) | Comparison of two methods of treatment for prostate cancer in terms of quality of life |
| 8 | May *et al.* (1995) | What is the impact of implantable cardioverter defibrillator implantation on quality of life? |
| 9 | Myken *et al.* (1995) | Do mechanical and porcine heart valve prostheses differ in terms of their effect on quality of life? |
| 10 | Phull *et al.* (1995) | What effect does the eradication of helicobacter pylori have on the quality of life of patients with chronic duodenal ulcer? |
| 11 | Pilpel *et al.*(1995) | What is the effect of growth hormone treatment on the quality of life of short-stature children? |

*Table 4.2* (Continued)

| Number | Authors | Question addressed |
|---|---|---|
| 12 | Rush *et al.* (1995) | What effect does ranitidine have on the quality of life of patients with gastro-oesophageal reflux? |
| 13 | Strauss *et al.* (1995) | Comparison of two methods of treatment for angina in terms of quality of life |
| 14 | Wijkstra *et al.* (1995) | Comparison of two patterns of rehabilitation in patients with chronic obstructive pulmonary disease |

disease (mentioned once each), patterns of rehabilitation for people with chronic obstructive pulmonary disease (mentioned once), and the treatment of children of short stature with growth hormone. Many of the interventions assessed in these studies are expensive and life-threatening, and their continuation would be threatened if it was consistently found that they have no beneficial impact on the quality of the lives of patients receiving them.

## Reliability, validity and other characteristics of scales used

Previous reviews of quality of life literature have found that studies use an enormous variety of questionnaires, interviews, psychometric tests, visual analogues and standardised tests to measure quality of life. For instance, Draper (1994) observed that twenty-five different scales were employed in a consecutive series of twenty studies. This pattern is repeated in the present sequence of studies, where the range of scales used includes a gastro-intestinal symptom scale devised by Visick (used in study 1), Karnofsky Performance Index (in studies 1 and 6), Spitzer Quality of Life Index (study 1), the SF-36 (studies 2 and 12), Living in a Supervised Home: a Questionnaire on Quality of Life (study 3), Psychosocial Adjustment to Illness Scale (PAIS) (study 4), the Mayo Clinic Post-

Laryngectomy Questionnaire (study 4), the Activities of Daily Vision Scale (study 5), the Functional Living Index: Cancer (study 7), Profile of Mood States (study 7), the Sickness Impact Profile (study 8), modified Gastro Intestinal Symptom Rating Scale (study 9), the McMaster Health Index Questionnaire (study 13), the Psychologic General Well Being Index (study 13), and the Chronic Respiratory Questionnaire (study 14). A number of researchers also reported the use of scales that were specifically designed for particular projects (studies 6, 7, 9, 11 and 12). Collectively, these scales employ a considerable number of variables as indicators of quality of life, as shown in Table 4.3.

*Table 4.3* Variables used to express quality of life in a series of fourteen outcome studies

| Study number | Variables |
| --- | --- |
| 1 | No details given by researchers |
| 2 | Physical functioning; social functioning; role limitations due to physical problems; role limitations due to emotional problems; pain, mental health, vitality, and perceptions of general health |
| 3 | Physical details of the home; access to community afforded by home; leisure opportunities available; community integration; routines within the home; resident education and training; staff behaviour, opportunities for residents to express choices and make decisions |
| 4 | Health attitudes; work or school; relationship with spouse; sexuality; family relationships other than spouse; hobbies and activities; psychological, medical and demographic data; methods used to cope with disability; perceptions of the treatment process; feelings about preparation for treatment; perceptions of laryngeal function |
| 5 | Ability to drive at night and during the day; vision disability; mental status; general health status; personal well-being; satisfaction with surgery; satisfaction with information, etc. |

*Table 4.3* (Continued)

| Study number | Variables |
| --- | --- |
| 6 | Cardiovascular symptoms; social support; satisfaction with life; general affect, well-being, etc. |
| 7 | Vocational, psychological, social and somatic areas of function; depression, anger, tension, confusion, fatigue and vigour; disease-specific symptoms such as bladder irritability, symptoms of urinary incontinence, sexual dysfunction and bowel dysfunction |
| 8 | Physical dimensions including ambulation, mobility, body care and movement; psychosocial issues including social interaction, communication, alertness and emotional behaviour; issues such as sleep and rest, eating, work, home management, recreation and pastimes |
| 9 | Overall quality of life; anxiety concerning the need for re-operation; thrombo-embolic events; anticoagulant and related bleeding; disturbance by valve sounds |
| 10 | Academic achievement; leisure activities; physical self-esteem; emotional self-esteem, relationships with peers and family members. |
| 11 | General health; use of anti-ulcer medication; dyspeptic symptoms; symptom severity; perceived general health |
| 12 | Physical functioning; social functioning; role limitations due to physical problems; role limitations due to emotional problems; pain, mental health, vitality, and perceptions of general health; a range of disease-specific issues such as diet, mental health, pain, sleep and social activity |
| 13 | Physical activities; mobility; self-care activities; communication; sexual function; mood; well-being; general health and vitality |
| 14 | Dyspnoea; fatigue; emotion; mastery |

There is no evidence that the medical researchers whose work is reviewed consider it a problem that such a profusion of scales is reported in the literature. Indeed, the argument is more often put that a range of scales is needed if we are to understand the impact that different diseases have on quality of life. For instance, Fayers and Jones (1983) argue that as, say, mastectomy for breast cancer produces different psychosocial problems from cytotoxic chemotherapy for lung cancer, it follows that different measures must be used if we are to understand the impact of each disease state on the quality of patients' lives.

Although this argument must clearly carry some weight, it does not, in my opinion, fully justify the use of such a large range of indicators for a single construct. One of the justifications offered for using quality of life as an outcome is that it enables different forms of treatment for a single condition to be evaluated, and a number of the studies reviewed here were conducted with this in mind (see for instance Buhl *et al.* 1995, Lim *et al.* 1995, Myken *et al.* 1995). However, several used different quality of life scales even though they were investigating closely related diseases or treatments. Thus, although Kumar *et al.* (1995), Strauss *et al.* (1995) and Myken *et al.* (1995) all report investigations into aspects of cardiovascular disease and its treatment, their use of differing quality of life measures means that direct comparison between the various interventions they describe is impossible.

Several of the papers reviewed employ quality of life measures that have not been used before but appear to have been developed by researchers specifically for the project (Freitas *et al.* 1995, Kumar *et al.* 1995, Myken *et al.* 1995, Pilpel *et al.* 1995). Sometimes these scales are combined with other well-known ones, but more commonly they are used alone. The justification for using such scales often seems to be that the researcher wishes to examine the quality of life of a particular patient group for the first time, and is unable to find a pre-existent scale. However, this practice also creates a number of difficulties, illustrated in the work of Freitas *et al.* (1995). Freitas and his colleagues were interested in discovering the effect of photorefractive keratectomy on the quality of their patients' lives. Patients recruited to the study were required to complete a scale designed to measure their functional status. This scale consisted of three subscales measuring physical, social and role functioning respectively. Each of these subscales contained one hundred individual items. The first problem relates to the enormous number of items in the scale. Quite apart from the difficulty that this imposes on patients, it suggests that the scale is poorly designed: one of the most popular and well-designed quality of life scales in current use, the SF-36, requires only thirty-six items to cover eight separate domains. In addition to completing this 300 item scale, the subjects were also required to complete three other scales: the Activities of Daily Vision Scale, the Symptom-Checklist 90 Revised, which contains ninety items, and the Cantril Self-Anchoring Striving Scale.

Additionally, most of the researchers failed to link their quality of life scale to an explicit statement of the meaning of quality of life in justification of the scale items used. Although the medical literature contains theoretical papers acknowledging that it is difficult to define quality of life (indeed, Hollenberg and his co-workers (1991) suggest that a satisfactory definition does not exist), the empirical literature tends to use the term in an unproblematic way.

Also, many researchers failed to offer any information about the conceptual basis, reliability, validity or psychometric properties of the scales they use, or, in the case of researcher-designed scales, about the procedure used to construct the instrument. Without this information, it is difficult to evaluate the quality of significance of the data produced by the research.

There is a close relationship between the reliability and the validity of psychometric and sociometric scales. An instrument is valid to the extent that it reflects the construct of interest to the researcher, and reliable if it does so in a consistent way (Reaves 1992). An instrument can be reliable without being valid, but validity always presupposes reliability (Walz *et al.* 1991). Bunge (1975) suggests that a valid quality of life scale will possess three characteristics:

1 an adequate definition of quality of life;
2 a range of indicators that are sensitive to and reflect variations in quality of life;
3 a theory that explains how changes in quality of life produce changes in the indicator.

Very few of the researchers discuss the validity of their instruments. Most appear to assume that their instruments have face validity, and some could claim content validity. However, none of the papers satisfy Bunge's criteria.

In summary, a proportion of the scales used in this research largely depend on face and content validity. This is associated with a lack of clarity about the nature of quality of life. In consequence, it is generally impossible to compare the findings of one study with those of another, although Najman and Levine (1981) have argued that this is one of the most important reasons for conducting research of this kind.

However, it is also possible to note positive trends in medical research to evaluate quality of life. The most striking is the emerging tendency of quality of life researchers to combine a disease-specific quality of life scale with a more general one in the same study. This is to be encouraged: the use of disease-specific scales may enable researchers to develop insights into the impact of particular disease states on quality of life, while using more broadly focused scales (such as the SF-36) may enable comparisons to be drawn between the impact of different therapies upon the quality of patients' lives.

## Research design

The studies employed a variety of research designs, described here according to the categories developed by Campbell and Stanley (1966).

The following researchers used retrospective designs: Myken *et al.* (1995), Kumar *et al.* (1995), and de Santo *et al.* (1995). From this point of view, the weakest study was probably that of Kumar and his colleagues. They wished to determine the quality of life of octogenarians after open heart surgery. Subjects' quality of life was measured some time after surgery, and they were asked to compare their post-surgical with their pre-surgical state retrospectively. This approach can be considered a variant of the one-shot case study. The finding of the study – that the intervention enhances quality of life – is arguably invalidated by the research design used, as the subjects might have given responses to please the researcher, who was also the clinician responsible for care. This danger is heightened because quality of life measures used involved patient self-assessment.

Phull *et al.* (1995), Freitas *et al.* (1995) and May *et al.* (1995) used the one-group, pre-test/post-test design. This is stronger than the retrospective design, as it enables the comparison of pre- and post-intervention measures. However, it also has a number of drawbacks. These include:

- history – the possibility that events other than the intervention may explain observed differences in pre-test and post-test scores;
- maturation – changes that occur naturally over time;
- testing – learning to answer the questions in a certain way;
- instrumentation – changes in the instrument over time.

The non-equivalent control group design also involves measurement before and after the intervention. Its principal weakness is that there is no way of knowing whether the groups are equivalent. This approach was taken by Pilpel *et al.* (1995) and Buhl *et al.* (1995).

The time-series design involves an intervention being made in the middle of a series of measurements. Campbell and Stanley (1966) consider that its biggest weakness is its failure to control history, and to this must be added the possibility of subjects attempting to please the researcher, particularly when self-assessment instruments are employed. This approach was taken by Freitas *et al.* (1995), Dagnan *et al.*(1995), Currie *et al.* (1995) and Lim *et al.* (1995).

Researchers were considered to have conducted a randomised clinical trial if they had randomly allocated their subjects to control and experimental groups, and measured before and after the intervention. In addition, some studies involved a degree of blindness. This approach, which provides the strongest evidence that an intervention has an impact on patients' quality of life, was taken by Rush *et al.* (1995), Wijkstra *et al.* (1995) and Strauss *et al.* (1995).

## Summary

In his discussion of the assessment of the impact of anti-hypertensive treatment on quality of life, Dahlof (1991) argues that it is extremely important that this type of study is methodologically faultless. He takes this to mean that the randomised, double-blind technique should be used wherever possible.

Although all medical or nursing interventions could not be assessed in this way, this review of fourteen outcome studies has shown that methodological weakness undermines the claims made by some researchers. For instance, the change which Kumar *et al.* claim to have detected could equally well be explained as the patients' desire to please the surgeon, or in a number of other ways. However, there has perhaps been a slight improvement in the general quality of research design in medical outcomes quality of life studies since Najman and Levine's survey of the literature in 1981. They found that only one study from a series of twenty-three could be classified as a randomised clinical trial, whereas the figure in this review is three from a series of fourteen.

In other aspects of the research, such as the definition of quality of life and the justification of indicators chosen, little advance seems to have been made. The great range of indicators chosen cannot be justified by the argument that different diseases impact upon quality of life in different ways; it is more likely to reflect an underlying inability to determine the nature of quality of life. As Najman and Levine (1981) argue, there has been a failure to derive an adequate conceptual understanding of what it means to have a better or worse quality of life. The argument made by Bunge in the context of social indicators research seems to apply here equally. He suggests that a better understanding of quality of life calls for more intense theoretical and methodological work rather than a simple increase in the amount of statistics. Here as elsewhere, he argues, data without ideas are sterile, or misleading, or both (Bunge 1975).

This chapter has focused on medical research into the quality of life, but it also has implications for nursing research and practice. Nurse researchers and their colleagues in clinical practice are becoming increasingly interested in the evaluation of nursing practice, and often attempt to relate particular nursing interventions to specific outcomes of care. There may be a strong temptation to use quality of life as an outcome, particularly when it is difficult to specify more concrete physical or psychological ones. This is not entirely inappropriate, but inadequacies in some of the medical literature reviewed above act as a caution against poorly conceived and conducted research. I suggest that before nurses embark on evaluative quality of life research they should follow the steps outlined in Box 4.2.

---

**Box 4.2** **Key points for using quality of life as an outcome**

● Nurse should be sure that they are using quality of life as an outcome not simply for the sake of it, but because they have a good reason to believe that it is the most appropriate outcome in this case.
● They should also take great care in the selection of scales. As we have seen, a great deal of medical research uses scales with poor or undisclosed psychometric properties. So many quality of life scales are now available that it should always be possible to find one that is both reliable and valid.
● It may be useful to use a global scale and a disease-specific one simultaneously.
● They should also ensure that the scales they choose are conceptually appropriate in that they are underpinned by a suitable definition of the quality of life.

# Chapter 5

# The social scientific approach to quality of life: positivism and its limits

The opening chapters have been concerned with three bodies of research that attempt to measure quality of life in various ways and for various purposes:

1 social indicators research, which represents the earliest systematic attempt to define and measure quality of life;
2 research into the quality adjusted life year, which advocates the concept of quality of life as a basis for making resource allocation decisions in the health service;
3 medical research which uses quality of life as an outcome to be measured in the evaluation of medical therapies.

These approaches to quality of life share a number of characteristics. Some of these relate to obvious issues such as the view that quality of life can be measured in principle. Others, however, are implicit and must be inferred from other evidence. In this chapter, we shall identify and examine some of these issues. Finally, the significance of the social scientific approach to quality of life for clinical nursing practice will be considered.

The most fundamental issue that links the social scientific approaches to quality of life is that they share a philosophical basis. The immediate purpose of describing the philosophical basis of social scientific quality of life research is first, to show that it exists, and second, to show that some of the assumptions embedded within it are questionable. Subsequently, it will be shown that it is possible to approach quality of life from other philosophical positions. One of these, philosophical hermeneutics, will be described later in the book.

At the root of social indicators, QALYs and medical outcomes research are two assumptions:

1   that quality of life is a 'social fact', or a rather concrete characteristic of people's lives;
2   that it is possible, at least in principle, to measure quality of life if the correct method is discovered and used.

These assumptions only make sense if one is prepared to adopt a philosophical framework grounded in positivism. I argue that a common belief, albeit implicitly held, in a positivist approach to social research is the most fundamental feature to link various social scientific approaches to quality of life.

Positivism refers to the view that the methods of the natural sciences can be legitimately applied to the study of the social world. Burrell and Morgan (1979) identify positivism as one of two great intellectual traditions which compete to define the nature of social reality, the other being antipositivism. Each tradition embodies assumptions about:

● ontology (what it means to be a human being and what is the nature of the social world);
● epistemology (what counts as valid knowledge)
● the relationship between the human being and the world;
● research methodology.

These are discussed below.

Of course, the debate about the nature of the social world is much more subtle and complex than appears to be the case when it is cast as an apparent choice between two polar extremes labelled positivism and antipositivism. However, it is perhaps true to say that many of the positions taken in this debate can be placed on a continuum between these two points, and that a good deal of progress has been made in our understanding of the social world as a result of dialogue between these two 'ideal types'.

## Positivist and antipositivist assumptions

The ontological debate concerns beliefs about the fundamental nature of human beings and their social world. Burrell and Morgan ask whether social reality is external to the individual in the same way that we presume the physical world is external, in that it exists 'out there', beyond the limits of one's body in an objective way, or whether it only exists as a product of cognitive processes and social interaction. Alternative positions in this debate are taken by the *realist*, who takes social reality to be an external phenomenon impinging on the consciousness of the individual from without, and the *nominalist*, who views social reality as a product of individual cognition and intersubjective reality.

The nominalist–realist debate gives rise to a second area of dispute, which concerns the nature of knowledge. Realists, who hold that the social world has a substance that is independent of the thoughts, beliefs and attitudes of individual people, argue that it is possible in principle to develop *objective* knowledge about it. A researcher who adopts this perspective is likely to employ methods akin to those of natural science and use various forms of observation to collect data. A nominalist, on the other hand, is more likely to adopt research strategies that will enable the social world to be viewed from the perspective of individual members of society in a rather *subjective* way. Nominalist research strategies are therefore likely to involve a degree of participation in the social world being studied.

The third set of assumptions concerns the relationship between human beings and 'their environment. On the one hand, Burrell and Morgan identify deterministic perspectives in social science, which view human behaviour as the mechanistic response to an external environment. These can be contrasted with voluntaristic accounts, which credit human beings with the possibility of free choice and independent action. In the former view, human beings and their experiences are regarded as products of the environment, conditioned by their external circumstances. This perspective can be contrasted with one which attributes to human beings a much more creative role: a perspective where 'free will' occupies the centre of the stage and the human being is regarded as the creator of his or her environment. These two extreme views of the relationship between human beings and their environment characterise a great philosophical debate between the advocates of *determinism* on the one hand and *voluntarism* on the other. Burrell and Morgan suggest that while there are social theories which adhere to each of these extremes, the assumptions of many social scientists are pitched somewhere between.

These three sets of assumptions have implications for the methods of social science. The *ideographic* approach emphasises the analysis of subjective accounts generated by 'getting inside' situations and involving oneself in the flow of everyday life. This is contrasted with *nomothetic* approaches, which emphasise systematic protocol and technique and the falsification of theory, as required by scientific rigour.

These groups of assumptions cluster together to define two competing intellectual traditions, as shown in Box 5.1.

---

***Box 5.1*** **Key points of positivism and antipositivism**

Positivism is defined by:
- a realist ontology;
- a positivist epistemology;
- a deterministic view of the relationship of the human being to the world;
- a nomothetic methodology.

In contrast, antipositivism:
- is nominalist in ontology;
- is antipositivist in epistemology;
- takes a voluntaristic view of the relationship of the human being to the world;
- favours ideographic methods.

---

Von Wright (1971) identifies three ideas that are central to positivism:

1   methodological monism, or the idea that scientific method is unified although the subject matter of scientific investigation is diverse;

2   the view that the exact natural sciences, in particular mathe-
    matical physics, set a standard against which the degree of
    development of all other forms of knowledge can be judged;
3   the view that explanation consists of the discovery of cause-
    and-effect relationships which can be expressed as laws and
    used to explain individual cases.

## Positivism and the social scientific approach

Several characteristics of social scientific quality of life research
suggest that it has a positivistic orientation to the social world.
These include the view that quality of life is a 'social fact', and the
practice of attempting to measure the level to which it is present in
people's lives.

First, let us examine the claim that social scientific approaches to
quality of life regard it as a 'social fact'. By this, I mean that each
body of research discussed above takes quality of life to be a rather
concrete characteristic of people's lives: a feature that appears to
exist in the same obvious and uncontentious way as sex, for example, or age appear to exist. Using Burrell and Morgan's definition of
positivism, this aspect of quality of life research indicates that a
realistic view of the social world is held.

It may seem that the assumption that quality of life is a social
fact is so obviously reasonable that no other position could logically be held. After all, if quality of life did not really exist in this
way, then why would so many eminent researchers behave as if it
did? It is worth remembering that the concept of quality of life, and
its use in literature, research and other settings, have a history. The
phrase was never used until the earlier part of the twentieth century
and, as we have seen, its use in research cannot be traced back
beyond the Second World War. It is entirely probable that if you
had used the phrase 'quality of life' in conversation in the pre-war
years, few people would have understood what it meant. This
begins to suggest that the concept is not quite as concrete as it
might appear: if it really were a factual characteristic of people's
lives, we might have expected scientists to have discovered it earlier.

Social scientific quality of life research demonstrates a number of
other links with positivism. Many researchers into quality of life in

the field of health employ techniques of social research borrowed from, or at least informed by, the methods of natural scientific disciplines, including medicine and experimental psychology. The research designs used are often based on the clinical trial, and scales are devised to measure the degree to which quality of life is present. These links are summarised in Box 5.2.

---

**Box 5.2 Links between the social scientific approach and positivism**

Social indicators, QALYs and medical outcomes research tend to a realistic view of human nature in that they believe quality of life to be a determinate characteristic of people. Their search for valid measurement tools confirms that they have a positivistic attitude to the nature of knowledge. Attempts to manipulate quality of life in various ways suggest a rather deterministic view of the relationship of person to environment, and the nomothetic approach is clearly evident in the nature of the research.

---

Careful analysis of published quality of life research shows that its implicit claims to objectivity and scientific rigour are, in fact, questionable. We have noted that social indicators research, QALYs and medical outcomes research all take place in a social context. For the social indicators researcher, this context is created by the need to influence policy: for the health economist who uses QALYs, resources are scarce and there is pressure to maximise efficiency; and for the medical researcher, it is professionally necessary to demonstrate that therapeutic interventions are effective. In each case, the social context has a bearing on the types of research question seen to be of interest and on the research methods used to answer them. This point was most clearly made in our discussion of QALYs, where it was shown that a change in the underlying assumptions that govern the collection and interpretation of data will have a direct influence on the answers that the research produces. This supports the view that quality of life data cannot be regarded as value-neutral, factual statements about people and the circumstances of their lives, because they are intimately associated with the researchers' perspectives and agendas.

A common assumption of social scientific approaches to quality of life is that quality of life is present or absent in some degree and can be measured if appropriate instruments and techniques are devised. In fact, difficulties in conceptualising and measuring the concept are common. They are most clearly evident in the medical literature, where it is relatively unusual to find operational definitions or explicit statements about the meaning of quality of life. The enormous range of variables used in the construction of measurement scales also suggests lack of conceptual clarity. Furthermore, medical researchers do not usually make explicit statements about the reliability and validity of the scales they use, and some researchers are too ready to use 'home-made' scales with unknown psychometric properties. The problems this involves were outlined in Chapter 4.

## Summary

Part I has examined three bodies of research-based literature into quality of life:

1   social indicators research;
2   QALYs;
3   medical research using quality of life as a measure of outcome.

Each of these approaches has been defined, research findings have been presented and difficulties discussed. It has been claimed that each approach is underpinned by a positivistic approach to the social world, and finally, various common difficulties have been identified. These include the effect of the social setting in which the research is conducted and problems of research design, conceptualisation and measurement.

# PART II
# Quality of life and nursing practice: philosophy and methods

# Introduction

In Part I, we found that most quality of life research is concerned with measuring the extent to which quality of life is present, with a view to:

- evaluating and generating social and political policy;
- making decisions about resource allocation in the health service;
- evaluating the outcome of medical treatment.

In Part II, the emphasis moves away from measurement and towards a discussion of the way in which the concept of quality of life can inform nursing practice. In Chapter 6, it is argued that the concept of quality of life has a useful contribution to make to clinical nursing practice; but to clarify the nature of this contribution, we need a degree of conceptual clarity about its meaning. It is argued too that useful alternatives exist to a concept of quality of life that is based on positivism, and philosophical hermeneutics is proposed as an alternative philosophical framework. In Chapter 7, a brief outline of hermeneutics is provided, and its implications for research method are discussed.

In summary, it will be shown that hermeneutics contributes to our understanding of quality of life in two ways:

1 by providing insights into the nature of human beings that challenge those of positivism;
2 by informing and justifying the research methods used in the empirical part of the study.

# Chapter 6

# The case for a nursing approach to quality of life

This chapter begins with the assumption that nurses have an interest in promoting the quality of life of their patients and clients. This immediately raises a number of challenging questions:

- How useful to nursing practice is the social scientific approach to quality of life?
- Are other approaches to quality of life available?
- How can nurses translate a highly conceptual notion such as quality of life into a series of practical steps that will promote the well-being of their patients and clients?

Social scientific approaches to quality of life are of limited usefulness to the clinical nurse. It is difficult to transfer concepts and ideas directly from the research setting to clinical nursing practice. Perhaps the chief reason is that the social scientific researcher is principally concerned with issues of operationalisation, measurement and research design, and has the ultimate goal in mind of generating information that will be used in decision making, resource allocation or evaluation. The clinical nurse is interested instead in creating systems of care and identifying professional activities which will safeguard and promote the quality of life of patients and clients. Clinical nurses will, it is true, in all probability be interested in research into quality of life published in the literature discussed above, and may wish to use published quality of life scales in the evaluation of their own work. However, the day-to-day clinical work of most nurses is more directly concerned with promoting quality of life than with the methods that can be used to measure it, and most of the social scientific literature on quality of life has little to contribute to this.

Before presenting an alternative to the positivistic, social scientific approach to quality of life, we need to begin by establishing and justifying the assumption that nurses have an interest in promoting and safeguarding the quality of the lives of their patients and clients. It may help us to understand the significance for practice of the concept of quality of life if we examine negative cases in which the quality of life of a group of people is clearly at risk. It is unfortunately the case that the literature of nursing and health contains many examples of abuse and cruelty. Many of these describe treatment given to disempowered older people or those with learning difficulties, and often arise in institutional settings. Three examples are given below, drawing upon the work of Robb (1967), the UKCC (1994) and Harman and Harman (1989).

## Three negative cases

One of the earliest accounts of cruel nursing care was given by Barbara Robb in 1967. Robb was one of the authors of a letter which appeared in *The Times* (Strabolgi *et al.* 1965) protesting about the practice, which was then common in general and mental hospitals, of stripping elderly patients of their spectacles, dentures, hearing aids and other civilised necessities, and of leaving them to 'vegetate in utter idleness'. The authors of the letter invited readers who had experience of these things to write to them giving details, and the resulting letters were compiled into the book *Sans Everything* (Robb 1967).

An extract is given below. It demonstrates the extent of the cruelty to which older people have, in the past, been subject, and stands as an extreme and obvious case of a situation in which quality of life is in jeopardy. However, it also provides a starting point from which to address the question: what is meant by quality of life? The extract was written by a male auxiliary nurse and describes practices in two large hospital wards in the north of England. The time period is from November 1964 to August 1965.

The patients feared the staff – especially the older, fully qualified charge nurses. Their fears were justified, as anyone present at 6.55am could vouch for, as they watched the charge nurse go into the assault armed with, for example, a short handled sweeping brush, and lay about him indiscriminately and with great ferocity. Bruises were commonplace, split eyebrows quite frequent. If the wound had to be stitched, it was always blamed on the assault of one patient on another.

The cruelty could be more refined than anything I have as yet described. Suppose for instance at meal-time a hungry patient brought his plate back for a second helping. Quite often it would then be deliberately heaped up in a revolting way with all the available scraps, until the food was piled to a height of perhaps 16 to 18 inches. The poor wretch was then 'stood over' until he had eaten so much it was a wonder the poor wretch didn't burst. And this took place not in Belsen, but in the north of England.

A patient complained to the visiting psychiatrist that the charge nurse had attempted to throttle him as he lay in bed. I had the story from the patient himself as he lay in bed, forced to remain there about a fortnight as a punishment. It appeared that the charge nurse, once the psychiatrist was safely out of the way, had merely repeated the process.

(Robb 1967:43–7)

It would be entirely misleading to suggest that nurses are uniquely responsible for the delivery of cruel treatment to older people. The report by Harman and Harman (1989) of the first ninety-six cases of the Registered Homes Tribunal shows that the problems can be much more widespread. Harman and Harman report a number of cases that they consider to be 'simply shocking': cases of neglect and callousness in which patients were verbally punished, bound in chairs, forced to hand over DHSS benefits under duress, left unattended for lengthy periods on commodes, and allowed to fall downstairs in unexplained circumstances.

Our final source shows that this problem should not simply be regarded as an historical one. The United Kingdom Central Council for Nursing, Midwifery and Health Visiting's occasional report (UKCC 1994) summarises the important issues arising from cases heard by the Professional Conduct Committee on the conduct of practitioners and standards of care in the nursing home sector. It presents statistics collated by the UKCC which show that professional misconduct cases in nursing homes constitute the largest single cause of complaint to the Council – almost 100 per cent greater than that for any other area of practice. Aspects of misconduct discussed in this report include physical abuse, administering excess doses of tranquillisers, administration of unprescribed medications, leaving residents in soiled beds, verbally abusing residents, and failing to promote the dignity of residents.

## The meaning of 'quality of life'

The three examples given above describe extreme and unusual circumstances in which older people have been subject to cruel and shocking treatment. Furthermore, and despite the fact that we are still not fully sure precisely what we mean by quality of life, it seems intuitively reasonable to suggest that each of these is discussing a situation in which the quality of life of a group of older people is in considerable jeopardy. We can make this claim because in each of the cases discussed, the treatment given is so obviously shocking.

But, we must not assume that the usefulness of the concept 'quality of life' is limited to discussions of the care of older people and others in residential care settings. It also seems quite reasonable to use the term to describe the intended outcome of other aspects of nursing care. Although it would be impossible to produce an exhaustive list, a catalogue of nursing functions whose goal is the restoration and maintenance of quality of life might well include:

● rehabilitation nursing;
● the management of pain;
● the behavioural management of phobias;
● the promotion of sleep.

There is, however, a danger that quality of life can be used to describe the goal of so many nursing functions that its meaning becomes quite lost. In order to avoid this, it is necessary to search for a degree of conceptual rigour and an answer to the question with which this book began: what precisely do we mean by quality of life?

Our search for meaning began with a critical review of the literature of social indicators, QALYs, and medical research using quality of life as an outcome. This review showed that each aspect of the quality of life literature contains common issues such as the persistence of the subjective–objective dichotomy and difficulties of conceptualisation and measurement, and it has been argued that the research focus of this work limits its significance for everyday nursing practice. Fortunately, the social scientific literature of quality of life does not exhaust the possibilities of the concept, as alternative approaches can be found in other scholarly traditions. One such body of literature is identified by Aiken (1982), who draws attention to a well-established philosophical approach which defines quality of life in terms of 'eudaemonia'. The roots of the eudaemonistic approach to quality of life lie in the work of Aristotle, and the term 'eudaemonia' has been variously explained in terms of happiness and human flourishing (Aiken 1982, Graham 1990). Aiken explains that philosophers in this tradition have typically tried to determine human essence, or to provide an answer to the question: what does it mean to be a human being? They have sought to define the 'good life' and to provide knowledge of both necessary and sufficient conditions for its attainment, and have been concerned with creating a social environment in which individuals can fulfil their potential.

The eudaemonistic approach to quality of life provides the starting point for certain ideas about the nature of quality of life and its promotion through nursing care, and these ideas form the focus of the rest of this book. Fundamentally, we are concerned with the question: what does it mean to be a human being? We shall see that various answers to this question can be found, each from a different scholarly tradition. There follows quite a short account of a particular approach derived from hermeneutics, a philosophical discipline principally concerned with the nature of understanding, but which also contains useful insights into the nature of human being. These insights form the organising framework for the rest of the book.

Subsequent chapters discuss particular aspects of quality of life from within the hermeneutical perspective. Chapter 9 concerns the importance of places and personal possessions, and Chapter 10 the meaning of individuality and choice. Both draw on previously published work and original research by this author. Chapter 11 discusses the application of these ideas to nursing practice. Here, the particular focus is on the organisation of nursing care for older people in residential settings other than their own homes.

# Chapter 7

# Hermeneutics: a philosophical basis for the study of quality of life

The eudaemonistic approach to quality of life is concerned with the nature of human being. In order to outline a eudaemonistic approach to quality of life that is significant for nursing practice, it is necessary to ask the three questions shown in Box 7.1

---

**Box 7.1 Key questions of the eudaemonistic approach**

- What is a human being?
- What are the circumstances in which human beings flourish?
- How as nurses can we bring about the circumstances in which human beings will flourish and avoid those in which they will not?

---

The remainder of this book provides an answer to these questions in outline.

What then do we mean when we use the term 'human being'? Perhaps the simplest approach would be to list a series of characteristics that human beings display. This has been done by a number of nurse theorists in the American tradition. For example, Dorothy Johnson regards the human being as a 'bio-psycho-social being who is a behavioral system with seven subsystems of behaviour' (Meleis 1991:274).

Although answers of this kind appear to have the benefit of simplicity, they tend also to be associated with certain problems. It is certainly possible to devise a list of human biological characteristics, but most if not all of these can also be found to some extent in other forms of life. As such, they cannot be regarded as definitive of human being. This difficulty becomes more pronounced in the case of the psychosocial aspects of human nature, as many items in a list of these characteristics would be culturally specific and not generalisable to all people.

Other nursing authors have sought to avoid such difficulties by making general and all-embracing statements. Rogers, for instance, defines the human being as 'an irreducible, four dimensional, negentropic energy field identified by pattern and manifesting characteristics which cannot be predicted from a knowledge of the parts' (Meleis 1991:314). This statement could also describe many forms of higher animal life, and in my opinion it is so diffuse as to lack significance in the world of professional practice.

It would be unwise for nurses wishing to gain insights into the nature of human being to neglect work done in other fields of scholarship, and here two types of resource can be found. First, views of the nature of human being are implicit in a number of general approaches or worldviews that inform and underpin work in several distinct areas of study. Positivism offers an example of such a worldview. As we saw in Chapter 5, it is a major intellectual tradition which offers an integrated account of the nature of the human being and the social world, and has implications for the ways in which we can understand that world. The founding fathers of positivism, such as Auguste Comte and J.S. Mill, were initially motivated not by a desire to pronounce on human nature but by a wish to discover and justify methods for creating scientifically valid knowledge about the social world. However, their approach has important implications for the way in which we view human nature, and for our understanding of the ways in which human beings interact with one another and with their environment.

Historically, a number of philosophers and social theorists have taken issue with positivism as an approach to understanding the social world. Collectively, their work constitutes an alternative intellectual tradition known, as discussed above, as antipositivism.

Philosophical hermeneutics is a discrete field of study within the antipositivist tradition.

The second type of resource is work done in individual fields of study under the theoretical umbrella of positivism, antipositivism or some other worldview. A useful philosophical review of seven specific theories of human nature implicit in work of this kind is provided by Stevenson (1987), who discusses Christianity and the works of Sigmund Freud, Konrad Lorenz, Karl Marx, B.F. Skinner and Plato.

Two significant twentieth-century scholars who made contributions of this type are Martin Heidegger and Hans-Georg Gadamer. Heidegger was an existentialist philosopher whose work specifically addressed the nature of human being, and in pursuing this question he also discussed the nature of understanding and interpretation. The focus of Gadamer's work was the nature of understanding, but once again his pursuit of this question led him to other important developments in philosophy. Both scholars made major contributions to hermeneutics

The philosophical hermeneutics of Heidegger and Gadamer provides the philosophical basis of the rest of this book. Hermeneutics was chosen because it gives an alternative approach to the positivism underpinning the social scientific approach to quality of life discussed above. The following account of hermeneutics begins with a discussion of the early phase of its development, principally in the work of Friedrich Schleiermacher and Wilhelm Dilthey. Heidegger's and Gadamer's contributions to hermeneutics are then discussed.

## An introduction to early hermeneutics

Hermeneutics is the branch of philosophy concerned with the nature of understanding. Its name can be traced back to Greek mythology. The Greek verb '*hermeneuein*' (to interpret) is taken from the name of Hermes, the deity whose function was to transmit messages from the gods to mortals, expressing them in such a way that they could be understood by human beings.

Early modern hermeneutics consisted of a body of practical techniques for solving problems in interpreting ancient documents such as the Bible, and secular texts whose meaning had become lost. The development of hermeneutics from a technical discipline to its modern configuration as a general philosophy of understanding is traced to the work of Friedrich Schleiermacher (1768–1834) (Ricoeur 1977).

Schleiermacher held the chair in Protestant theology at the University of Berlin between 1810 and 1834. One of his most important contributions to the development of hermeneutical theory was his recognition that understanding is a 'circular' phenomenon in which a simultaneous comprehension of the whole and the parts is required. Palmer (1969) offers a succinct explanation of the 'hermeneutical circle', summarised in Box 7.2.

---

***Box 7.2* The hermeneutical circle**

Palmer says that we understand something by comparing it to something we already know. In this process the whole, and the parts of which that whole is composed, play complementary roles. A sentence, for instance, is made up of a sequence of words. Both the whole (the sentence) and the parts of which it is constructed (the individual words) have a role to play. We understand the meaning of an individual word by seeing it in reference to the whole of the sentence; reciprocally, the meaning of the whole sentence depends on the meaning of individual words A kind of dialogue takes place between the whole and the part, in which each gives the other meaning.

---

Palmer considers that Schleiermacher's contribution to hermeneutics marks a turning point in the development of the discipline, suggesting that his goal of a general hermeneutics as the art of understanding, and his early account of the hermeneutical circle, are of particular importance. Schleiermacher's work also provided a platform for later philosophers who wished to oppose the development of positivism as an approach to understanding the social world.

One such was Wilhelm Dilthey (1833–1911). Dilthey's contribution to hermeneutics can best be understood in the context of the market place of ideas which characterised the Europe of the late eighteenth and early nineteenth centuries. Dilthey worked in the shadow of Immanuel Kant, who in his three 'critiques' had examined the nature of knowledge in the mathematical and natural sciences, and the role played by the human mind in the construction of that knowledge. Dilthey's particular field of interest was not the natural sciences, but a group of disciplines which he called the '*Geisteswissenschaften*', including history, sociology and anthropology. Dilthey's goal was to describe the methods through which valid knowledge could be created in these disciplines.

In the early part of the nineteenth century, the debate about the nature of the social world and the methods that could appropriately be used to understand it was dominated by the positivism of Auguste Comte. Comte was impressed by the spectacular advances of science and technology (Giddens 1976), and he argued that just as laws had been found to explain the interaction of elements in nature, so they could be found for the interaction of people in society.

Dilthey was dissatisfied with Comte's positivism as an approach to understanding the social life of human beings. Dilthey argued that there are fundamental differences between the subject matter and goals of the natural and social sciences. To him, it was apparent that the natural sciences take as their subject matter the many phenomena which constitute the physical world, and that their goals are to describe these and then to formulate laws to account for the relationships between them: the natural sciences are explanatory sciences.

Dilthey argued that the type of knowledge afforded by the cultural sciences was qualitatively different. Our knowledge of human history and culture could never be direct, but is always derived from the study of a group of phenomena which he called 'objectifications of life'. Wilson (1989) refers to these phenomena as 'cultural achievements', including human productions such as works of art, social movements, political ideologies, texts, dances, constitutions and laws, political forms such as socialism, democracy and fascism, and languages, religions, customs and traditions.

Dilthey believed that the explanatory procedures of the natural sciences are of little use in helping one to grasp the individuality and meaning of cultural expressions; the proper goal of the cultural sciences is to understand these cultural expressions, and the forms of life that they represent. For him, understanding was essentially an intuitive process made possible by shared humanity.

The development of early hermeneutics is summarised in Box 7.3.

---

**Box 7.3  Summary of early hermeneutics**

The early phase of hermeneutics saw it develop from a set of techniques used to understand the meaning of obscure secular and religious texts, to a philosophical discipline whose goal was to understand the phenomenon of understanding itself. It began a critical dialogue with positivism about the nature of the social world, the methods through which that world might be understood, and the type of knowledge that would result. For Dilthey, the methods of natural science could not be applied directly to the human sciences because of differences in their subject matter: whereas the physical sciences were concerned with developing universal laws in order to explain the interaction of elements, the human sciences sought to understand expressions of culture in terms of categories drawn from life itself. Understanding was essentially an intuitive phenomenon, and was possible because each cultural achievement, having been created by human beings, could in principle be understood by human beings.

---

## Martin Heidegger: the hermeneutical dimension of being

The first substantial development in twentieth-century hermeneutical theory came in 1926 with the publication of Heidegger's difficult work, *Being and Time*. Dreyfus (1991) suggests that part of

Heidegger's purpose in writing this book was to work out a fresh analysis of what it means to be a human being.

Heidegger denied that the nature of human being could ever be reduced to a fixed or determinate list of characteristics. Seeking to explain his understanding of this nature, he developed and applied the concepts of interpretation and understanding, derived from the hermeneutical tradition of Schleiermacher and Dilthey. In addition, he used the flexibility of the German language to invent new terminology to express his ideas. His well-known concept of 'being in the world' was created in this way.

Heidegger argued that our understanding of the nature of human being is distorted by certain powerful ideas handed down from a previous generation of philosophers, including René Descartes, whose work was influential in justifying many of the assumptions on which positivism is based. Descartes (1986) had based his account of understanding on the premise that the mind and the body were distinct and separate entities. The mind ('*res cogitans*', or ' thinking substance') existed in the dimension of time, whereas the body ('*res extensa*' or 'extensive substance') was physical in nature and occupied three-dimensional space.

Descartes's dichotomy between mind and body created a problem: how is it possible for the mind to know anything about a physical world to which it can never have direct access? Descartes argued that the mind had to build up its understanding of the world by compiling impressions that it received by way of the sensory mechanism of the body. True knowledge could be said to exist when the contents of the mind corresponded with some state of affairs in the external world, but unfortunately there was always the possibility that impressions gained about the world might be flawed or mistaken.

How, then, is it possible to be sure of facts or to gain true knowledge? For Descartes, the search for truth necessarily involved minimising the effect of subjective influences and seeing things in an objective way. Bernstein (1983) suggests that the Cartesian tradition conformed to the basic conviction that there must be some permanent matrix or framework which is free from the distorting influences of history, culture and subjectivity, and to which we can ultimately appeal in determining the nature of rationality, truth, reality, goodness and rightness. Descartes expressed these views in his search for an 'Archimedean point'. Archimedes, who explored the nature of levers, had said that all he needed in order to move the earth was a place to stand and, presumably, a big enough lever. Descartes's search for an Archimedean point represents his search for a place to stand that was free from distorting influences of all kinds.

Generations of philosophers and methodologists have followed Descartes in assuming that if they could find a method of freeing themselves from the distorting influences of history and society, they would be able to perceive the world in its pristine reality and thereby claim certainty in knowledge. For Edmund Husserl, for instance, Descartes's Archimedean point could be achieved through phenomenological reduction. Bauman (1978) explains that this method requires the individual to cut himself or herself off from all historical and social entanglements so that consciousness, liberated from the world, can grasp meaning in its true and necessary essence. At the other end of the methodological spectrum, the experimental psychologist Kerlinger (1973) considers that truth can most nearly be approximated if the scientific method is rigorously applied.

Heidegger's views on the nature of human being, the relationship of the human being to the world, and the nature of knowledge are radically opposed to those of the Cartesian tradition. He begins by denying Descartes's fundamental distinction between mind and body, and re-evaluating their relationship to the world. Through the notion of 'being in the world', Heidegger asserts that the relationship of human being and world is one of necessary interdependence. The notion of being in the world has two aspects, expressed in Jean-Paul Sartre's comment that 'without the world there is no self-hood, no person; without self-hood, without the person, there is no world' (Macquarrie 1972:81).

The suggestion that 'world' depends on human being should be taken to imply not that the material world relies for its existence on the minds that perceive it, but rather that human concern and involvement serve to integrate diverse phenomena, organising and imposing a framework of coherence upon them, and thereby constituting them as 'world'. Macquarrie comments that Heidegger's use of 'world' is related to the sense of the Greek word '*kosmos*', which means not only 'world' but 'order', and implies the organisation and unity brought about by personal involvement (Macquarrie 1972:79).

We hint at Heidegger's use of 'world' when we speak of 'the world of work' or 'the world of politics'. He is implying that the world we inhabit is not simply a neutral environment in which, by chance, we can be found; but that it consists of an integrated and coherent system of meanings, objects, values and purposes which are structured and organised by, and expressive of, human purposes and goals.

The notion of being-in-the-world also expresses Heidegger's argument that 'world' is essential for human being. Material objects such as tools and equipment are not neutral artefacts. As they are put to everyday use by the human beings who participate in the shared social practices of a particular culture, they come to carry a burden of meaning, and form a part of the 'symbolically structured environment' (Bourdieu 1977:87) within which daily life is lived. In my daily work, for instance, I am employed as a university lecturer. As I write, I am surrounded by books, papers and equipment for writing. At my side is a computer that can be used for statistical analysis, writing or searching the Internet; and my academic robes hang in a bag beside the filing cabinet. These artefacts are equipment that enable me to do my job, but their significance extends beyond their practical function. The books on the shelves behind me are useful not only for the information that they contain – in fact, I rarely look at them – but because they act as signifiers of my work and role. My academic robes have no function as practical items of clothing, but are worn on graduation days because of the symbolism and meaning invested in them. Collectively, these objects and meanings constitute my professional world.

Being-in-the-world forms the background to Heidegger's discussion of 'interpretation'. This is related to the special, non-colloquial sense he gives to the concept of 'existence'. His comment that 'the essence of *Dasein* [the human being] lies in its existence' (Heidegger 1962:42) is not to be taken as indicating the obvious fact that each human being is real in that he or she occupies a point in space. As

Cooper (1992) explains, Heidegger's technical use of the word 'exist' draws on its derivation from Greek and Latin words which mean 'to stand out from', and refers to the belief that a person is always already 'beyond' or 'ahead of' whatever properties characterise her or him at a given time. Cooper argues that no complete account can be given of a human being without reference to what she or he is in the process of becoming, the projects and intentions that she or he is striving to realise, and the terms in which she or he makes sense of her or his present condition. As Heidegger puts it, the human being is always '*unterwegs*', (on the way).

The notion of existence is closely related to the role of interpretation in the process of human being. Dreyfus (1991) argues that both human beings and their cultural institutions have existence as their 'way of being'. To exist, he suggests, is to take a stand on what is essential about one's being, and to be defined by that stand. He argues that the human being is what, in its social activity, it interprets itself to be. Dreyfus denies that human beings already have some specific nature, and suggests that there is no reason to believe that we are essentially rational animals, creatures of God, organisms with built-in needs, sexual beings or complex computers. Human beings, he contends, can interpret themselves in any of these ways and many more, but to be human is not to be essentially any of them. Human being is essentially simply self-interpreting.

Logically, the mode of being which Heidegger calls existence, and the related activity of interpretation, are possible because the human being is at all times faced with a range of possible courses of action: a 'space of possibilities' closes off certain courses of action while maintaining others as 'live options'. This space of possibilities depends on the physical, social and historical situation of the individual – upon his or her 'being-in-the-world' – but it never serves to commit a person's actions in a deterministic way. As Guignon (1992) explains, our human agency is always located in a specific cultural context that provides the pool of possibilities from which we draw our concrete identities.

Benner and Wrubel's (1989) discussion of the nature of caring provides a useful illustration. They point out that although a person caring for a loved one with a serious illness often appears courageous to someone who is not involved, the care-giver does not feel courageous because the option of not caring does not present itself as viable.

Heidegger's discussion of being-in-the-world, interpretation and existence have implications for the ways in which we understand. His account of the nature of understanding is radically different from Descartes's. Heidegger rejects the view that understanding involves extracting ourselves from the world, arguing on the contrary that it is only possible because we have our being-in-the-world. He asserts that there are three non-cognitive pre-conditions of understanding, which he calls the 'fore-structure'. These three elements are summarised by Dreyfus (1980:10, 1991:198) as follows:

1  *Vorhabe* (fore-having). The *Vorhabe* is the totality of cultural practices which constitute the taken-for-granted background which circumscribes our possibilities for understanding and determines possible ways of questioning.
2  *Vorsicht* (foresight). *Vorsicht* implies that our understanding is mediated by the vocabulary or conceptual scheme which we bring to bear on a problem.
3  *Vorgriff* (fore-conception). *Vorgriff* relates to the fact that in each act of understanding the investigator has an expectation of what will be discovered.

In the practice of science, the *Vorhabe* is what Kuhn (1970) calls the 'disciplinary matrix', – that is, the skills and concepts which a student acquires in becoming a scientist, which enable him or her to determine what the scientifically relevant facts are. The *Vorsicht* relates to the theoretical framework of an investigation; and the *Vorgriff* is the particular hypothesis in question.

Heidegger's contribution is summarised in Box 7.4.

## Hans-Georg Gadamer: understanding as the fusion of horizons

The work of Heidegger's friend and pupil Hans-Georg Gadamer recapitulates elements of the work of Schleiermacher, Dilthey and others, but he was particularly influenced by Heidegger. In *Truth and Method*, Gadamer's most important work, elements and

**Box 7.4 Summary of Heidegger's contribution**

Heidegger moved hermeneutics beyond Dilthey's concern with the methodological concerns of the human sciences by showing that understanding and interpretation are characteristics of human being. As Kisiel (1969) comments, for Heidegger, the movement of interpretation is no longer an encounter between an interpreter and a difficult text, but one between human existence and the unique historical situation in which it occurs. Both the 'text' and the 'author' of earlier hermeneutical theories are drawn into this larger context.

themes from each of these writers are gathered up and synthesised into a new whole, as the writer works out his intention to 'discover what is common to all modes of understanding' (Gadamer 1975:xix).

Gadamer's task is reminiscent of Schleiermacher's aim of developing a general hermeneutics; but although Gadamer shares with Schleiermacher the view that hermeneutics is, or ought to be, a general discipline, he does not make it his purpose to inform the methodology of the human sciences, or to develop an art or technique for the interpretation of texts. He is concerned with a more fundamental question: how is understanding possible, not only in the humanities but in the whole of the human's experience of the world (Palmer 1969)? Gadamer rejected the view, held since the Enlightenment, that truth is to be identified exclusively with the products of the scientific method. As Page (1991) comments, the title of his work (*Truth and Method*) announces Gadamer's intention of undermining the orthodox view that the positive sciences are the ultimate paradigm of cognitive success, and that scientific method is wholly adequate to all of the truth.

Gadamer's critique of the Cartesian tradition extends that which Heidegger had begun in *Being and Time*. According to the tradition, the scholar who espouses objective truth must recognise that:

● he or she holds certain presuppositions and prejudices;

- these presuppositions and prejudices have the power to distort his or her understanding;
- their effect can be minimised through the use of a method.

The method may be Husserl's phenomenological reduction, which enables the scholar to put his or her presuppositions 'in brackets' in order to discount their effect; it may be the scientific method, or some other. Method is necessary because, as Peters (1974) comments, presuppositions for the natural scientist are like 'lice in the hair': they are to be eliminated, for in his work, the ideal scientific thinker believes she or he must become a blank slate, a purely open mind onto which the data of her or his research can inscribe unbiased knowledge.

Gadamer rejects these arguments. It is his view that the prejudices which a person holds are derived from his or her historical situation; and he argues that far from being the enemy of understanding, prejudice constitutes its necessary precondition (Gadamer 1975). (Where Gadamer uses the word 'prejudice', some of his commentators substitute 'presupposition'. The two terms will be used interchangeably here.)

Gadamer seeks to reclaim the concept of prejudice from negative connotations, which he traces back to the Enlightenment. The word was originally derived from two Latin words: '*pre*' (before), and '*judex*' (a judge). It therefore simply refers to a judgement which has already been made. For Gadamer, our prejudices cannot be divided from the historical nature of our being: from the fact that each of us is historically as well as socially situated. He believes it is less accurate to say that history belongs to us than that we belong to it. He suggests that long before we understand ourselves through the process of self-examination, we do so in a self-evident way in the family, society and state in which we live. He describes the focus of subjectivity as a distorting mirror, and suggests that the self-awareness of the individual is only a flickering in the closed circuits of historical life. For Gadamer, the prejudices of the individual, far more than his or her judgements, constitute the historical reality of his or her being.

Gadamer's analysis of the role played by prejudice in understanding draws on Heidegger's theory of the fore-structure of understanding. Gadamer argues that the prejudices which tradition hands down to a person constitute his or her 'situation'. Our prejudices create a standpoint that simultaneously creates and limits the possibility of vision. This standpoint can be understood if we liken it to the horizon. The horizon is the range of vision that includes everything that can be seen from a particular vantage point, defining what we can see, and also constituting that beyond which it is impossible to see.

The concept of horizon provides Gadamer with a powerful metaphor which he uses to explain the process of understanding. For Gadamer, both the scholar and the text which is the object of study exist within horizons whose boundaries are determined by their historical situation. Gadamer is critical of earlier hermeneutical theorists such as Schleiermacher and Dilthey for underestimating the role which the historicality of the interpreter plays in the process of understanding (Linge 1976). Understanding does not occur as the scholar steps out of his or her own horizon and into that of the text, for that would not be possible; but neither does it involve the relentless superimposition of the prejudices of the scholar upon the text. Rather, understanding is the result of the formation of a comprehensive horizon in which the limited horizons of text and interpreter are fused together into a common view of the subject matter with which both are concerned – the meaning. Thus, understanding can be defined as the fusion of the horizons of scholar and text.

Conversation offers a good model of the way in which understanding occurs. Palmer (1987) considers that in a true conversation, one person does not simply ask questions of the other in order to discover what the other thinks: this would be not conversation but interrogation. Equally, however, we do not say that two people are in dialogue when one is haranguing the other without listening to the response. True conversation demands a quality of openness from both participants: an attempt by each to discover what the other is saying, and a preparedness from each to place her or his own prejudices at risk through openness to what the other has to say.

If this model is applied to historical understanding, it:

- shows that truth in history is not discovered by attempting to recreate the mental processes of those whose texts, words and deeds we have received;

● invalidates attempts to make definitive pronouncements about the meaning of historical events.

Although we need to discover the standpoint and horizon of the other person for her or his ideas to become intelligible to us, this does not necessarily imply that we agree with her or him. Two important aspects of Gadamer's hermeneutics deserve final emphasis:

1  Gadamer's argument that prejudice plays a necessary role in understanding does not imply that the range of a person's prejudice is fixed, that his or her prejudices are all equal in validity, or even that they are all defensible. However, the person who seeks to understand the past will find that his or her understanding of the present is also enhanced, and that the prejudices which constitute his or her own horizon will come more clearly into view. Gadamer suggests that we should test all our prejudices. He argues that the historical movement of human life consists in the fact that it is never utterly bound to one standpoint, and hence can never have a truly closed horizon. Horizons change for the person who is moving.

2  Gadamer's approach obviates the possibility of arriving at a definitive or canonical interpretation of a given text. Particular interpretations cannot claim objectivity because each is the product of the interaction of the horizon of the text with that of the interpreter. Consequently the meaning of a text will vary in different historical periods (Hekman 1984). This means not that the process of interpretation is an arbitrary one, or that competing interpretations are of equal validity, but that judgements of the validity of a particular interpretation of a text will, like the interpretation itself, be influenced by the horizon within which they occur (Bernstein 1983).

The hermeneutical tradition is summarised in Box 7.5.

# Hermeneutics and qualitative research methodology

Many practical and theoretical disciplines have explored the implications of hermeneutical philosophy for their research methods.

**Box 7.5 Summary of the hermeneutical tradition**

The hermeneutical tradition provides an account of the nature of human being and the interrelationship of human being and world that stands in opposition to the assumptions of the positivist tradition, on which the social scientific approach to quality of life is based. The human being is regarded less as a fixed set of properties than as an interpretative process, which takes place at a point whose boundaries are defined by history, culture and place, and which is exemplified and displayed by shared meaning. Understanding does not arise as we step out of our world, but is made possible by a horizon of meaning whose existence depends on our being in the world.

Before the 1970s, discussions of hermeneutics were most commonly found in such disciplines as continental philosophy, theology, and literary criticism (Thompson 1991), and there has since been increasing reference to hermeneutics in the methodological literature of the social sciences. This discusses hermeneutics as a philosophy that redefines the scope and nature of the social sciences (see, for instance, Bauman 1978, Giddens 1976), and supports an approach to social research which focuses on meaning and understanding in context. Thompson (1991) suggests that this methodological literature is part of a movement among practitioners and scholars in applied disciplines and the social sciences who are becoming dissatisfied with positivism as an adequate philosophical grounding, and notes that as a consequence of the steady growth of interest in the 1980s, hermeneutics has emerged as a philosophy whose relevance extends beyond the humanities to the social sciences, practice disciplines, and even the natural sciences themselves.

The primary literature of hermeneutics does not discuss method (Barrett and Sloan 1988). Neither Heidegger nor Gadamer was a social scientist, and in the introduction to *Truth and Method*, Gadamer explicitly states that his purpose is not to describe a method of interpretation, but to discover what is common to all modes of understanding. Many nursing scholars misunderstand this point, and describe a 'hermeneutic method' in such a way that one would imagine them to be following the methodological prescriptions of Heidegger and Gadamer themselves. However, although hermeneutics does not offer methodological tools on a par with, for example, statistical analysis, it clearly does have implications for research method (Hekman 1986) and by extension for nursing research. Some of these implications are now explored.

Hekman (1984, 1986) recognises a dichotomy in the methodological literature of the social sciences. Its objectivist or positivist pole received early expression from J.S. Mill, who argued that the behaviour of human beings in the social context does not differ methodologically from the movement of physical objects. Hekman contends that positivist research entails replacing the social actor's own understanding of his or her actions with the social scientist's precise, unambiguous concepts, and with the analysis of data according to the universal rules of logic and scientific method, focusing particularly on causality. This approach is deemed to avoid the subjectivism entailed by reference to social actors' understanding of their actions. (See Bunge 1993 for a contemporary exposition.)

Hekman distinguishes the positivist approach from an 'interpretative' school whose position, although less easy to define, is characterised by agreement on two points:

1  The methodology of the social sciences must be regarded as different from that of the natural sciences, because social action can only be defined by reference to the subjective meanings of social actors.
2  The purpose of the social sciences is to understand social action rather than to subsume it under a universal law of causality.

Hekman suggests that the methodological debate between these two schools has reached deadlock, and argues that Gadamer's philosophical hermeneutics offers a way of transcending this problem. She argues that his notion of understanding as the fusion of horizons, when applied to social research, avoids the problems inherent in both the subjectivist and objectivist approaches, and reminds us that for Gadamer, meaning is neither located in the subjective intention of the author or actor, nor produced by the interpretative methods of the scholar. Rather, understanding occurs as the horizon of the scholar intersects or fuses with that of the text. In practical terms, Hekman contends that the notion of understanding as the fusion of horizons permits the scholar to respect and retain the perspective of the research participant, and simultaneously to approach the data or focus of enquiry from the perspective offered by a nominated theoretical position. In describing the interaction between the horizons of interpreter and text, Hekman draws on Gadamer's metaphor of understanding as a dialogical process. This, she believes, legitimises the imposition of the observer's conceptual scheme without denying the constitutive role of the social actors' concepts (Hekman 1984).

Similarly, Thompson (1991) suggests that hermeneutic philosophy emphasises the social and historical nature of enquiry, and shows that understanding cannot be separated from the social interests and standpoints that we assume as the result of being cultural agents. Hermeneutics, she argues, shows us that human understanding is limited and conditioned by our social interests, values, language, concepts, time and history, and helps us to understand that the decisions made in the process of doing research are value laden and interest bound. Wachterhauser (1986) agrees, arguing that hermeneutical thinkers can be characterised by their concern to resist the idea of the human intellect as a wordless and timeless source of insight. He suggests that human understanding is never 'without words' and never 'outside of time'. On the contrary, human understanding is distinctive because it always occurs in the context of some evolving linguistic framework that has been worked out over time in terms of a historically conditioned set of concerns and practices. Wachterhauser suggests that language and history are always both conditions and limits of understanding.

Hermeneutical emphasis on the social, historical and contextual nature of understanding is reflected in this book in the assumption that we cannot discover ahistorical features of quality of life that can be isolated, described, measured and manipulated. However, the hermeneutical view of understanding as social, historical and contextual also warns against a form of radical subjectivism, bordering on solipsism, that suggests quality of life is a completely private and idiosyncratic affair. Consequently, while the hermeneutical basis of this research suggests that care must be taken when extrapolating the findings to some wider population, it also implies that there is no reason in principle why they might not inform the situation of others, particularly if the findings can be supported by evidence drawn from the broader philosophical, theoretical and empirical literature.

Some specific implications of hermeneutics for the conduct of qualitative research are discussed in the next section.

## Hermeneutics and the conduct and analysis of qualitative interviews

The author conducted research to discover the meaning of quality of life for a number of older people living in residential accommodation apart from their own homes, and for their professional carers. The principal method used was qualitative interview. Hermeneutics has considerable implications for the conduct and interpretation of qualitative interviews. These implications will now be discussed.

Kvale (1985) suggests that the qualitative interview is a particularly suitable method of data collection for hermeneutical research, because it implies a hermeneutical mode of understanding in which people can describe their world, opinions and acts in their own words, and subjects can organise their own description, emphasising what they themselves find important.

Honey (1987) also believes there is an intrinsic relationship between hermeneutics and the research interview. She argues that both are driven by the interplay between 'belief' and 'scepticism'. On the one hand, she suggests, hermeneutics is animated by 'faith', by a willingness to accept what is given at face value. On the other hand, she recognises that hermeneutics has traditionally sought to uncover hidden and obscure meaning. She refers to this as 'the hermeneutics of suspicion'.

The tension between the hermeneutics of faith and that of suspicion is apparent during the interview process, where the researcher's willingness to let the participants speak is complemented by strategies designed to expose contradictions and uncover deeper levels of meaning. It is also apparent during the analytical process, where the goal of presenting a clear account of the informant's views is matched by an attempt to discover the assumptions upon which those views rest, and to highlight the conflict that sometimes exists between the rhetoric and the reality of nursing practice.

Practical considerations in the conduct of the interviews, such as sampling and interview technique, will be discussed in the next chapter. This one will close with a consideration of the implications of hermeneutics for the interpretation and analysis of qualitative research interviews.

## The guiding principles of analysis

Hermeneutical researchers commonly describe analysis as a sequential process of several stages. Thus, Benner *et al.* (1992) describe a five-stage analytical process, and Rather (1992) and Diekelmann (1992) both describe seven-stage ones.

This discussion rejects the process approach because it comes too close to reducing hermeneutics to a method, and would therefore contravene Gadamer's work. Also, a sequential account would not reflect the complex dialogical interplay between the horizons of the text and interpreter which is central to hermeneutical analysis.

Despite these problems, it is clearly important to explain the relationship between the raw data and the findings that constitute the next three chapters. The following account reflects the work of Miles and Huberman (1994), who suggest that qualitative analysis is a non-linear activity consisting of three concurrent activities:

1  *Data reduction* is the process of selecting, focusing, simplifying, abstracting and transforming the data as it appears in transcriptions or field notes.
2  *Data display* consists of organising and presenting the data so that conclusions can be drawn by a transparent process.
3  *Conclusion drawing/verification* consists of confirming the validity of the conclusions through argument, replication of the findings in another data set, placing the conclusions in the context of theory, or in various other ways.

The following account discusses the principles that guided analysis, but does not reduce that analytical activity to a linear process.

## Principle 1: Transcribed interviews can be treated as text for analysis

The first stage in hermeneutical analysis of qualitative interviews is to transcribe the interviews, interleave them with plain paper for notes, and bind them in a suitable folder. They can then be regarded as text for the purpose of hermeneutical analysis. The social scientific and practical disciplines that draw on hermeneutics commonly regard documents and artefacts of various kinds as texts or text analogues in precisely this way. For instance, Kurz and Nunley (1994) describe the archaeological remains of an ancient city as a text analogue for the purposes of hermeneutical analysis.

Honey (1987) argues that a transcription is like a conventional text because it is a work:

- It consists of a structured whole that cannot be reduced to its individual components.
- It is produced according to a series of rules that define its literary genre (research interview).
- It is characterised by the style resulting from the interaction of interviewer and interviewee.

Kvale (1985) notes that the text is not pre-given in qualitative research, but is created by the joint efforts of researcher and participants. It bears the mark of the researcher's theoretical framework, sampling decisions, choice of questions, interviewing strategy, and guiding research question. Consequently, the interviewer is co-author of the text. (In this respect, the research text varies in kind from the texts that are the traditional focus of the hermeneutical approach.)

## Principle 2: Interpretation is not an arbitrary activity

It is recognised in hermeneutics that a single text is open to many different interpretations, each of which may be valid in principle.

This is because the meaning of a text is not simply defined in terms of the subjective intentions of its author but is the outcome of the fusion of the horizons of text and interpreter. Consequently, interpretations that proceed from different perspectives may be equally acceptable. As Eagleton (1983) argues, the meaning of a literary work is never exhausted by the intentions of its author, and as it passes from one cultural or historical context to another, new meanings may be derived from it which were never anticipated by its author or contemporary audience.

This means that the validity of a particular interpretation of qualitative research data is not necessarily a function of its reproducibility, although this is the mark of validity in natural science and positivist social science. Kvale (1985) supports this point, arguing that if the principle of the legitimate plurality of interpretations is accepted, it becomes meaningless to impose conventional standards of validity.

Although the principle of understanding as the fusion of horizons may lead us to reject the idea that there is a single correct interpretation of a text, it does not follow that all interpretations are equally valid. Hekman (1984) suggests that horizons are particular vantage points which, although they encompass a range, are also exclusive. She does not reject the notion of validity *per se*: her point is that interpretations are not arbitrary, and that criteria must exist by which they can be evaluated. Two such criteria are suggested in Box 7.6.

The validity of the interpretation of my own data text (see Part III) is defended, first, on the grounds that it is the result of a systematic approach. Kvale (1985) points to the danger of reading a complex text as the devil reads the Bible: in other words, of selecting passages that support the interpreter's preferred view, and neglecting those that suggest a contrary one. It is important to counter this danger by ensuring that the interpretation draws on every part of the text.

Furthermore, the researchers' understanding of the participants can be validated during the interview process by techniques such as focusing and clarifying, as described below. Kvale (1985) suggests that interpretation is concurrent with, rather than distinct from, data collection. The validity of the interpretation is supported if it corresponds with the findings of empirical literature from a number of disciplines. This literature is summarised and integrated into the findings, as presented below. Finally, the interpretation is supported by multiple extracts from the text.

---

**Box 7.6 Criteria for evaluating interpretations**

- A valid interpretation will be defensible. As Kvale (1985) comments, what matters is to formulate as explicitly as possible the evidence and arguments applied in an interpretation, in order for it to be testable by other readers. Giorgi (1975) suggests that it is necessary to show whether a reader adopting the viewpoint articulated by the researcher can also see what the researcher saw, whether or not the reader agrees with it. Ricoeur (1981) agrees. He suggests that it is always possible to arbitrate for or against various interpretations, and that the researcher's task is to show that the given interpretation is more reasonable than any of the limited number of other constructions that could have been presented.
- Hekman (1984) suggests that interpretations may be evaluated in terms of the common understandings of the linguistic community and in our critical examination of and openness to tradition, and specifically by their conformity to the horizon from within which the interpretation was conducted.

---

## Principle 3: Interpretation involves description of the text

For the sake of clarity, the next sections discuss interpretation as if it contained two elements: a descriptive phase that proceeds from within the horizon of meaning of the text; and a later one in which the text is approached from the interpreter's horizon of meaning. In reality, the practice of interpretation involves continuous dialectical movement between the two horizons. Consequently, the effect of the interpreter's horizon is apparent during description of the text; and conversely, the nature of the text modifies the researcher's understanding of her or his own theoretical perspective.

There is a degree of consensus that hermeneutical analysis involves a descriptive element. Hekman (1984) suggests that an interpretation should clarify the horizon of the text: it should give an account of the participants' view of the phenomenon under study, and should clarify the assumptions, beliefs and views that constitute their perspective. Benner (1985) and Bryckzynski (1989) support this view.

Kvale (1985) notes that transcribed interviews are often vague and repetitious, with many digressions, and that they generally contain a lot of 'noise'. He suggests that identifying the essential meanings of a text may require an extended process of condensing, although he recognises that what originally appears as noise may eventually yield important information. It is for this reason that early attempts to 'clean up' the text should be avoided, and the interview transcribed in its entirety.

The descriptive component of this interpretation is based on a systematic categorisation. This process may begin with:

- line-by-line analysis of the data (Strauss 1987);
- an initial comprehension of the whole text (Jones 1985).

The principle of the hermeneutical circle asserts that both the parts and the whole are important in understanding. Analysis must therefore function at both levels, giving an adequate account of the entire text, and building this account by identifying discrete units of meaning. The first analytical task is therefore to develop a sense of the whole of the text. This is accomplished by reading through it several times. It is then necessary to move from the whole to the parts. This phase involves developing and defining basic units of meaning known as 'categories'. A category can be defined as 'A bit of data that presents an intelligible and coherent point which is in some sense self-sufficient' (Dey 1993:94). Categorisation of the data involves two interrelated processes:

1 identifying the categories within the text (also known as constructing a category list);
2 collating every instance of each category in the text.

There is a view in qualitative research that the process of categorisation is an inductive activity in which categories 'emerge' from the data (Glaser and Strauss 1967). Dey is implicitly critical of this approach, arguing that there is never a single set of categories 'waiting' to be discovered, but that there are many different ways of 'seeing' the data (Dey 1993:110), each of which will reflect the researcher's perspective or horizon of meaning.

The process is rather fluid in nature. When the text is first read, an initial and rather tentative set of category titles is affixed to the data. When the whole text has been categorised in this way, it may become apparent that some of the category titles represented the idiosyncratic view of a single informant, that others are rather trivial in nature, and that a third group represents issues that were discussed by many of the informants and were conceptually significant. The category list is then adjusted as certain provisional category names are deleted, while the portion of text to which they referred is subsumed under a more appropriate title.

Although every part of the text is scrutinised during categorisation, certain portions may not be subsumed within a category. The most common reason for excluding a part of the text is that it represented 'noise'. Other portions that might have been classified in principle may be excluded because their content is irrelevant in terms of the research question.

After the category list has been developed, the entire text is re-read, and each instance of every category is collated. Subsequent analysis draws on the data as reorganised into categories. Categories may then be explored for major themes, structures and processes, and areas of agreement, disagreement, contradiction and tension may be discovered.

## Principle 4: Interpretation involves the fusion of the horizons of the interpreter and the text

Hermeneutical interpretation involves but is not limited to systematic description of the text within the terms of its own horizon. One of its strengths is that it permits the scholar to respect and retain the perspective of the research participants, and simultaneously to approach the text from a different horizon of meaning.

The effect of the historical perspective is present in any study in various issues, such as the background to the project, the research question, methodological decisions and the approach to data collection, all of which have their impact on the final shape of the text. Hekman's suggestion that the interpreter's horizon is also constituted by a specific ideological perspective is taken up by Thompson (1991). She argues that hermeneutical researchers must deal explicitly with their own interpretative theories and should understand that the use of these provides them with a specific ideological perspective. She discusses as an example the work of Melosh (1982), who used the theory of professionalisation as an interpretative background that provided a specific orientation to 'the facts' in her historical study of professionalisation in nursing. Thus, Hekman (1986) and Thompson (1991) broadly support Dey's (1993) suggestion that analysis involves a dialectic between ideas and the data.

In the case of my own research, presented below, philosophical hermeneutics provided the ideological orientation. Hermeneutics offers a contribution to the debate about the nature of quality of life. Benner (1985) draws on this as she suggests that quality of life might be conceptualised as the quality of being. Her approach is congruent with a well-established philosophical tradition that defines quality of life in terms of eudaemonia, as discussed in Chapter 6. The ideological perspective adopted during this study, which forms part of my interpretative horizon, draws on the contribution that Heidegger's ontology makes to our understanding of the nature of the human being, and the study's outcome is intended to contribute to the eudaemonistic approach to quality of life.

During the descriptive phase of interpretation, the scholar's ideological perspective acts as a lens that enables him or her to see certain categories in the text. In the present case, for instance, Heidegger's notion of being-in-the-world, which represents the idea that the physical world is saturated with meaning, sensitised me to numerous instances where physical artefacts such as personal possessions are valued more for their meaning than for their usefulness.

In other cases, the process of categorisation was less self-consciously informed by the researcher's perspective, and category titles were derived from the vocabulary used by the informant.

## Summary

Chapter 7 has suggested that philosophical hermeneutics offers the foundations of a eudaemonistic approach to the quality of life with significant implications for nursing practice. The chapter began with three questions:

- What is a human being?
- What are the circumstances in which human beings flourish?
- How as nurses can we bring about the circumstances in which human beings will flourish and avoid those in which they will not?

We have seen that a number of philosophical traditions have implications for our understanding of the nature of human beings. One of the most important and influential of these traditions is positivism. This underpins scientific approaches to the human being such as behavioural psychology, and has also influenced the work of a number of nursing scholars.

Our brief exploration of the work of Schleiermacher, Dilthey, Heidegger and Gadamer has shown that hermeneutics has developed through dialogue and in opposition to the positivist tradition. In hermeneutics, the human being is regarded not as a creature characterised by a fixed set of properties, but as the product of an interpretative process which takes place in the context of history, culture and place.

Hermeneutical philosophy is relevant to this project because it contributes to our understanding of the nature of human beings. It is doubly relevant, however, because it informs the practice of qualitative research, and the chapter has closed with a discussion of principles that guide the methods of data collection and analysis that can be used in a hermeneutical study.

# PART III

# Quality of life: a nursing perspective

# Introduction

This part takes the first steps towards the development of a eudaemonistic theory of quality of life: a theory that draws upon
hermeneutics to offer an account of what it means to be a human
being, and identifies ways in which professional nurses can promote the quality of the lives of their patients and clients. It is
implicit that we cannot construct a universally valid account of
quality of life. According to the hermeneutical tradition of
Heidegger and Gadamer, the nature of human being can never be
expressed or described as a set of principles valid at all times and in
all places. Instead, we must elaborate the notion of a eudaemonistic approach to quality of life by working it out in the context of
the lives of the specific group of people who contributed to this
study. It may, however, be valid to generalise to other populations
of people, particularly if it can be shown that they share important
cultural and social characteristics with the original group. Also,
the following is not an exhaustive account of the features that make
for a life of quality for older people living in hospitals, nursing
homes and other settings apart from their own homes.

The following discussion draws upon three sources of evidence,
integrating them in the way discussed in the previous chapter. These
are:

1  the literature of philosophical hermeneutics, which, as we have
   seen, offers an integrated and coherent account of what it
   means to be a human being, how human beings are related to
   their physical and social worlds, and what counts as valid
   knowledge of those worlds. Hermeneutics constitutes the chapter's conceptual framework. Particular use is made of ideas
   developed by Heidegger and described in *Being and Time*;
2  data derived from research interviews held with a number of
   elderly people living in a range of health care settings apart

from their own homes. These interviews were transcribed and taken as data for qualitative analysis in the manner described in Chapter 7;

3 empirical work by other researchers, reported in the published literature.

Chapter 8 describes a number of practical steps taken in the conduct of the research, and Chapters 9–11 present some of the findings. Chapter 9 considers the importance of places and personal possessions for the quality of older people's lives, and Chapter 10 explores the importance of choice. In Chapter 11, there is a discussion of how nursing care can promote the quality of the lives of older people in hospital wards, nursing homes and other similar settings. Chapter 12 considers some of the wider implications for nursing practice of the contents of this book.

# Chapter 8
# Research decisions

The goals of the research described in this part were:

- to develop a concept of quality of life with the power to explain the significance of the violations of the rights and dignity of older people that sometimes occur in institutional care;
- to describe some of the positive steps that practitioners take to promote the quality of life of their patients and clients.

The study was undertaken at various hospitals in a single health authority in the north of England. The purpose of this chapter is to describe practical matters, such as the sampling techniques and interview strategies used.

## Sampling

Sampling decisions reflected the need to identify people who could discuss the meaning of quality of life for older people and describe practices and situations which both enhanced and impaired that quality. Accordingly, two major groups of research participants were chosen: older people currently receiving nursing care, and members of occupational groups responsible for the organisation and delivery of that care. Sampling decisions were modified by the inclusion of participants from each of the many types of hospital facility available in the health authority where the research was conducted. The size of the sample was also shaped by two factors:

1 this need to include participants from each facility;
2 redundancy of data, which occurred when the pool of ideas and practices described by the research participants appeared to be exhausted.

Seven hospitals in the health authority had long-stay facilities for elderly people. Hospital A had a number of wards classified as 'psycho-geriatric'; Hospitals B, C, D, E, and F had a mixture of rehabilitation wards and long-stay facilities; and Hospital G was a busy district general hospital with a number of acute 'geriatric' wards, and some long-stay places. The selection of Hospitals A, C, E, F and G provided a mixture of acute, long-stay and 'psycho-geriatric' facilities.

A staged form of quota sampling (Cohen and Manion 1989) was used to select individuals for interview, with the hospital ward as the basic sampling unit. One ward was selected from each of the hospitals chosen, with the assistance of the hospital nursing managers, who provided access to the weekly meetings of the ward sisters. At these meetings, the purpose and nature of the research project were explained, and all who wished to participate were invited to volunteer. In this way, five wards were chosen, one from each hospital. An element of self-selection was inescapable because it would not have been possible to involve wards without the permission and goodwill of the sister.

A number of older people were then selected from each of these five wards. It was felt inappropriate to delegate this selection to ward staff, who might have been reluctant to choose patients they considered to be confused or difficult. In principle, any patient was considered to be eligible for the study whose name appeared on the ward list. Patients were selected from the list according to the categories shown in Box 8.1.

---

**Box 8.1 Categories used for selecting patients**

- patients of both sexes;
- patients who had, in the opinion of the staff, a reasonable prospect of discharge home in the near future and those for whom this prospect was remote;
- some patients classified by the staff as confused and some not;
- most importantly, patients who were willing to be interviewed for the study.

In total, fourteen elderly patients were selected in this way and agreed to participate in the study.

It is clear that the staff who manage and deliver hospital care can influence the quality of the lives of elderly patients. As the ward sisters probably have the greatest potential influence, we interviewed more of them than any other staff group. We invited the ward sister/charge nurse from each ward from which patients had been selected to participate in the study, and eleven accepted. We also included two district nursing sisters, one social worker, one occupational therapist, one physiotherapist, one nurse manager, one staff nurse and one physician.

## Interview technique

The technique of ethnographic interview (Martin *et al*. 1984) was used to collect data. This type of interview is not a free conversation, but it does not follow a highly structured list of pre-determined questions. The interviewer's task is to structure the encounter so that the informant can give a full and clear account of his or her ideas. As the interviewer cannot avoid influencing the conversation, the goal is to make the exchange of information as comfortable as possible while remaining focused on understanding the participant's meanings, and questions are worded to give the interviewee an opportunity to confirm or correct the interviewer's understanding of his or her meaning. The interview was not structured according to a fixed list of questions, but certain 'stem questions' were held in mind, as shown in Box 8.2.

These questions were used to get the interview started while retaining the focus on quality of life. The subsequent strategy was to respond to the issues contained in the participant's answer to these opening questions, and to explore them in greater depth. The following example of an opening question is taken from the interview with Sister A:

*Researcher*: So . . . the topic is quality of life. Can you tell me what the phrase means to you . . . in connection with elderly people? There is no such thing as a wrong answer . . . I just want to know what you think.

***Box 8.2* Stem questions for structuring interviews**

- What do you understand by the phrase 'quality of life'?
- Can you suggest other terms for 'quality of life'?
- (To staff) What do you do in order to promote the quality of the lives of the patients on this ward?
- (To older people) How do the staff help to promote your quality of life?
- (To staff) If you could do one thing to improve the quality of the lives of the patients on this ward, what would it be?
- (To older people) If one thing could be done to promote the quality of your life, what would it be?

As each interview developed, the techniques of focusing, clarifying, reflecting and summarising that are described in the context of the helping interview by Egan (1986) and Connor *et al.* (1984) were employed.

Data were analysed according to the principles discussed in Chapter 7.

# Chapter 9

# Being at home: the relationship of places and personal possessions to quality of life

This chapter is concerned with the roles that places play in the lives of older people, and with the significance of physical objects such as personal possessions and clothing. It is argued that the ways in which nurses think of places and physical objects are commonly guided by scientific disciplines such as psychology and physiology. The scientific approach regards places and personal possessions as aspects of 'the environment', and tends to focus more on their objective characteristics than on their meanings and significance. It is argued that the Heideggerian perspective encourages us to think in terms of meaning and significance, and research is reviewed which sees places and possessions in these terms. Particular attention is paid to:

- the phenomenon of attachment to place;
- the meaning of personal possessions and the roles they play in the well-being of the older person;
- the importance and significance of clothing.

## The theoretical perspective

Many nurse theorists, particularly those in the American tradition, claim that 'the environment' is one of the central concerns of the theory and practice of nursing (Fawcett 1989). Typically, their view of the relationship between person and environment is informed by the scientific disciplines of physiology and psychology. For instance, King (1981) claims that the internal environment of human beings transforms energy to enable them to adjust to continuous external environmental changes, while Roy (1984) suggests that it is made up of all conditions, circumstances and influences surrounding and affecting the development and behaviour of persons or groups.

When the British nursing literature explores the phenomenon of environment, it also tends to be preoccupied with objective characteristics. For example, when Cormack (1990:3) praises nurse managers 'who are sufficiently enlightened and flexible to provide equipment, furniture, decoration, or wall covering that is varied, domestic, and otherwise non-clinical and non-institutional' in order to 'present the illusion of home rather than hospital', he misses the point that 'home' is valued for much more than its non-institutional appearance. Furthermore, the importance that Cormack attaches to the physical characteristics of the environment is not justified by research evidence, which shows that the level of satisfaction people express with their dwellings is only weakly correlated with objective characteristics such as the number of rooms and the state of structural repair (Campbell *et al.* 1976, O'Bryant 1982).

The scientific approach encourages us to consider the environment in terms of observable, measurable and objective characteristics, such as the distance between two points. Such an approach is, of course, extremely useful in a number of ways: in geography, for instance, it helps us to produce maps which specify the distance between places, and the type of terrain that separates them. However, although it is clear that the scientific conceptualisation of the person as existing in an environment is useful in some circumstances, it is a highly specialised approach that does not correspond with or inform the human being's normal experience of the physical world. Where science expresses direction in terms relative to the fixed points of the compass, the normal, everyday human experience is of direction and distance relative to the disposition of the body. We take the human body as reference point when we describe things as being on the left or the right, behind or before, or up and down. Phrases that describe distance in terms of human activities are also common, as when we speak of something 'a stone's throw away'. Thus, where the scientist expresses distance in standard units of length, the everyday experience is of a spatial world whose meaning is expressed in terms relating to human concerns and activities. This experience of space presupposes the ownership of a human body and frequently expresses values and meanings. In several cultures, that which is above is both morally and physically superior to that which is below; to be seated at the right hand is a special sign of favour; and regrettable episodes in life are 'put behind one' (Tuan 1977, Dovey 1978).

Scholars from various disciplines have been critical of a tendency to examine the environment in purely 'objective' or scientific terms. Some of these writers have been self-consciously influenced by Heidegger's writing, while the work of others corresponds with his approach. For instance, Ley (1977:500) criticises social geography for becoming overly concerned with the categorisation of 'landscape facts . . . sprung loose' from their everyday context in the human world, resulting in the transition 'from a science of man in place to a science of phenomena', and preparing the way for a 'scientism which ultimately abstracted place to a geometry of space and reduced man to a pallid entrepreneurial figure'. Ley argues for an approach to geography that recognises the subjective as well as the objective, and the adoption of a philosophical underpinning that embraces both object and subject, fact and value. Heidegger's insights into the day-to-day experience of space have prompted scholars from fields as diverse as environmental psychology (Seamon 1982), sociology (Agnew and Duncan 1989), architecture (Lukermann 1961), gerontology (Rubinstein 1987, 1989) and anthropology (Rowles 1981, 1983a, 1983b) to explore the phenomenon of place as a locus of meaning. For instance, Relph (1976) has suggested that the identity of places is constituted by three fundamental components which, although irreducible one to the other, are inseparably interwoven into our experience of places. These are:

1 the static physical setting;
2 the range of activities with which each place is associated;
3 the range of meanings that places often hold for people.

## The phenomenon of attachment to place

Rowles (1983a, 1983b) conducted an ethnographic of the elderly residents of Colton, a small American town in economic decline.

He was particularly interested in the fact that his elderly subjects were deeply attached to Colton, the place in which many of them had lived for most of their lives, and he wanted to examine the ways in which this sense of attachment arose and the forms that it took. He developed a theory of 'insideness' to explain the phenomenon of attachment, and this offers a useful theoretical principle that enables us to understand aspects of the experience of older people in hospital and nursing homes settings, as interviewed for this study. In this section, reference is made to existential insideness, physical insideness, social insideness, and autobiographical insideness.

## Existential insideness

Every hospitalised elderly person who was interviewed during the course of this research expressed a desire to return home or regretted that this was no longer possible. This is seen in the simple response of Mrs A:

*Researcher*: Where would you rather be then?
*Mrs. A*: At home.

Later in her interview she was asked:

*Researcher*: What sort of things do you think about?
*Mrs A*: I think about am I going to stay here all the time or am I going to go home. They never mention about me going home.
*Researcher*: They don't say anything?
*Mrs A*: No
*Researcher*: Not at all?
*Mrs A*: No, nothing about going home.
*Researcher*: Do you talk about it?
*Mrs A*: Yes. I say to them, 'When am I going home?', but they say 'All in good time.'

Indeed, the desire to return home was even expressed by a woman whose early brain-failure made much of the rest of her conversation meaningless:

*Researcher*: Where would you rather be then?

*Mrs B*: At home! (said very positively).
*Researcher*: Why?
*Mrs B*: 'Cos it's too new
*Researcher*: Why would you rather be at home?
*Mrs B*: Because . . . I like . . . it's just . . . it's just . . .

Some of the elderly people interviewed clearly felt that the desire to return home was so self-evidently 'normal' that its justification was neither necessary nor possible, while others were able to explain or illustrate the reason for their attachment to home. The following extract from an interview held with Mrs C serves as a point of departure for an explanation of the meaning of home for older people that draws both upon the data and the empirical literature:

*Mrs C*: Where would I rather be? There's nowhere else really. I'd rather be at home in my own home, but it's impossible really because I can't see for one thing. I did manage, you know.
*Researcher*: Why would you rather be at home?
*Mrs C*: At home? Well, I'd be in the house I lived in, and I'd be satisfied.

This passage illustrates something of the complexity of the concept of home. As the word is used here, it can be interpreted in three different ways:

1  Mrs C's mention of 'my own home' refers to a specific place, either a house or flat, which has its own postal address.
2  Her wish to be 'in my own home' is expressive of her desire to return to that place.
3  To be 'at home in my own home' reveals the sense of attachment to place that is so characteristic of the experience of home.

Relph reserves the term 'existential insideness' for the experience of knowing implicitly that *this* is the place to which you belong. He defines this as the experience that people have when they are at home and in their own town or region: when they know the place and its people and are known and accepted there. He suggests that existential insideness characterises the deep and complete sense of identity with a place that is at the foundation of the concept of 'place'.

Further evidence of existential insideness can be found elsewhere in the data, where Mr D's comment that: 'What me and the wife would like to do is go back to the flat, put on the fire, and do the usual things,' gives a sense of his desire to return to a place that is valued for its familiarity. In contrast, Mrs C's remark that: 'You have to be content [here in hospital even though] it's another world,' indicates her profound sense of displacement.

## Physical insideness

*Mrs B*: One thing I don't like is you have to keep asking for the commode all the time when you can't go yourself. I've been trying to find it myself this morning. I don't know where it is. I don't know my way around yet. If I can go on my own I'll be happy. I won't have to ring anybody.

This quotation demonstrates the innate sense of familiarity with place that Rowles (1983a) calls 'physical insideness'. The elderly person's knowledge of the home environment does not simply exist in a cognitive form. In his study of the process of attachment to place, Rowles (1983a) used the term 'body awareness' to describe the finding that his elderly subjects had internalised a sense of the pathways they traversed during the rhythm and routine of their daily lives. He found that over the years, each old person had developed an intimate familiarity with environmental barriers, slippery places, and pathways affording frequent physical supports to compensate for an unsteady gait.

Rowles's notion of body awareness serves as a specific instance of Heidegger's more general concept of 'readiness-to-hand'. This occurs where an item of equipment in use 'is transparent or unnoticed, an extension of the body and the action' (Benner and Wrubel 1989:412). It describes skilled, habitual performance in familiar circumstances, and is characteristic of many of our un-reflective dealings with the physical world, such as the use of equipment and tools. When we use a hammer, for instance, we are not interested in its properties in the detached and objective manner of the scientist; rather, our focus is on the task of hammering.

For the older person, the familiar environment of the home is ready-to-hand in this way. If older people are removed from the place to which they are accustomed and which for them is ready-to-hand, their capacity for independence may be impaired. Rather than facilitating the processes and activities of daily life, the unfamiliar environment becomes an obstacle that gets in the way. Heidegger calls this state 'un-readiness-to-hand':

> In our dealings with the world of our concern, the un-ready-to-hand can be encountered not only in the sense of that which is unusable or simply missing, but as something which is not missing at all and not unusable, but which 'stands in the way' of our concern. That to which our concern refuses to turn, that for which it has 'no time', is something un-ready-to-hand in the manner of what does not belong here, of what as yet has not been attended to. Anything which is un-ready-to-hand in this way is disturbing to us, and enables us to see the obstinacy of that with which we must concern ourselves in the first instance before we do anything else.
>
> (Heidegger 1962:103)

Un-readiness-to-hand precisely describes the situation of Mrs B, in the quotation with which this section began. She finds herself in an unfamiliar environment, and rather than facilitating her concern – which is to use the commode – the environment 'stands in the way'. This is disturbing to her and, to paraphrase Heidegger, the accomplishment of environmental familiarity becomes that with which she must concern herself before she does anything else.

## Social insideness

*Researcher*: What are your plans from the hospital?
*Mrs F*: Why, to go home as soon as I can.
*Researcher*: That's your plan?
*Mrs F*: Yes, and probably one of my nieces will pop in every day.
    And my granddaughter with the two children, she pops in after

school, you know, she fetches the children from school and pops in to see me. If I write down something I wanted, then she'll see I get it.

Rowles (1983b) suggested that the intimacy of physical insideness was supplemented by a sense of social insideness, stemming from integration in the social fabric of a local age peer group, and constituting a supportive milieu with shared norms of behaviour and a common value system. In their study of the local sense of place as experienced in north-east England, Taylor and Townsend (1976) also identified a social aspect to the link between person and place; the familiarity and friendliness of the local area were particularly important.

For many older people, home is the fulcrum of the social dimension to their lives, because it is a place that provides them with the opportunities and means to socialise, entertain, be close to and maintain contact with family and friends (Rutman and Freedman 1988). For some, the home may represent a reservoir of family history and a link between past and future generations.

There is a temporal dimension to the link between person and place: it takes time to develop a network of friends. Rowles found that many of the individuals who constituted the social network of his research subjects were age peers, with whom relationships had been developed over a lifetime of shared experience made possible by residential proximity. For this reason, length of residence and a history of shared social experiences tend to strengthen attachment to place, whereas a history of mobility tends to reduce it (Taylor and Townsend 1976).

## Autobiographical insideness

*Mrs G*: My plan is to go home. My daughter has asked me to live with her but I don't want to. I love my home, even though it's just a corporation house and it's too big. I've lived there for fifty-four years.

As part of his research, Rowles (1983a) drove elderly people about the town so that they could show him the places that were particularly evocative of past friendships, the memories of childhood, and other important events in their lives. 'Autobiographical insideness' describes the sense of attachment that links person to place through the memory of important events in one's personal history.

This section has established that home is important to the older people who were interviewed. In the next section, various important characteristics of home are identified. Priority is given to the data from my own study, but other research is integrated into the discussion as and when relevant.

## Home as a locus of autonomy

Some older people said that home was important because it was a place where they were free to make choices:

*Researcher*: But what do you like about being at home, though?
*Mrs C*: Being able to please yourself. Freedom of being able to choose what you do and what you eat. You see, you can't do that in hospital.

Similarly, Mr H said that he would rather be at home than in hospital because then he could do what he wanted to do: go out, watch TV, go to bed when he wanted, and so forth; and Mrs G, explaining why she missed her home, said it was the place where she could do what she liked: turn the lights on or off, watch the TV, talk to her neighbours. This gave her a sense of independence. It is interesting to note the mundane nature of the choices that were valued by these older people.

The theme of home as a place where choice is maximally available is examined in the literature. Furby (1978) identified control as an explanatory variable for the acquisition of property; and in a study of older people who had chosen to relocate to age-segregated, rent-subsidised apartments, Rutman and Freedman (1988) found that responses from 57 per cent of the relocated group and 72 per cent of the waiting-list group suggested that home was valued because it gave the opportunity of personal autonomy.

Some writers explain the claim that the home is valued as a locus of autonomy in terms of a theory of territoriality. Porteous (1976) suggests that the human being shares with many animal species a tendency to assert exclusive jurisdiction over physical space. The territorial boundary, which may exist in either a physical or a symbolic form, demarcates a zone to which access may be controlled by an individual or a social group. Porteous suggests that control of territory is maintained by two major means: personalisation of space, and defence of space; and that territorial ownership bestows a range of satisfactions that includes identity and security. He suggests that there is a particular link between personalisation and identity, and argues that the placement and display of personal objects in the home constitute an important display of the self.

Porteous also suggests that the defence of space through the control of territorial boundaries bestows a sense of security. Whereas animals tend to use scent or excreta to mark the extent of their ranges, human territorial boundaries are marked in culturally specific ways. Porteous notes the difference between the rigid demarcation between public and private domains expressed in the high wall surrounding the Muslim dwelling, and the much less defensible open plan of many western dwellings. He argues that the importance of territorial boundaries is illustrated by the 'sanctity of the threshold', and the rituals involved in entering the home of another, such as knocking on the door.

In this section, we have seen that home is important because it may offer opportunities for personal control. Two particular forms of control have been explored:

1  Control of territorial boundaries has been linked to a sense of security.
2  Personalisation of the environment has been linked to the expression of identity.

In the next section, the role of personal objects as a medium for self-expression will be examined in more detail. It will be suggested not only that personal possessions are important as signs of the self, but that they also have a role to play in the constitution and maintenance of the self. Other roles for personal possessions will be identified too.

## The meaning of personal possessions

At interview, older people sometimes said that they wanted to go home because home was the place where their personal possessions were to be found. In the following discussion, the significance of personal objects for older people will be explored.

*Mrs B*: When I get better I want to go home. Everybody likes their own home. I miss my telly and all that.
*Researcher*: What do you like about your own home?
*Mrs B*: My telly.

Mrs I, another interviewee, also introduced the idea that home is important because certain things are to be found there:

*Researcher*: What do you do at home?
*Mrs I*: We have a cassette with loads of opera, operatic and classical music on it, and I look at television if there's a good film on. I read a lot, lots of books. And of course I have friends come in. We can chat and that. In the summer when the flowers are out, roses and that, I can go in there among the roses. Yes, in the fresh air.

Finally, Mrs J felt that no one could be really happy in hospital because people were not surrounded by their own things.

Rochberg-Halton (1984) describes two theoretical traditions in which personal objects have been taken as significant:

1   environmental studies;
2   semiology, or the study of symbols and signs.

These are examined below.

The environmentalist tends to emphasise the physical characteristics of material artefacts. This is the position taken by Cormack (1990:3), who praised nurse managers for decorating their wards in a domestic style 'in order to present the illusion of home rather than hospital'. We have already noted Cormack's failure to attend to research that demonstrates a weak correlation between the level of satisfaction that people express with their dwellings and observable characteristics such as the number of rooms and the state of structural repair. As Taylor and Townsend (1976:104) report, there is not necessarily anything about the nature of the physical or built environment which influences people's sense of belonging to it. At interview, Sister K made a related point:

'Some people are happy at home, in appalling home circumstances – perhaps in back-to-back houses with no heating, in dirty surroundings – and they're happy. That's their life, and they're happy with that life.'

The second theoretical tradition that Rochberg-Halton describes is semiology, which is rooted in Freudian psychoanalysis. An example is found in the work of Winnicott (1951), who elaborates the concept of the transitional object to refer to external things that are not distinguished completely from the individual's own person. According to Winnicott, transitional objects are those things that initially take the place of the breast before the individual has gained a sense of the distinctness of self and other. Winnicott also includes more subliminal versions of transitional objects that are applicable to the later stages of the development of the self, but that retain the underlying psychological meaning of the breast-substitute. The idea of the transitional object is taken up by Sherman and Newman (1977), who suggest that objects could help elderly people to move from independent to institutional living, and note a positive correlation between the ownership of cherished personal possessions in residential care, and life satisfaction score.

In his comparative critique of the traditions of environmental studies and semiology, Rochberg-Halton (1984) says that each displays a tendency to ignore or deny what the other assumes. While environmentalists have often failed to appreciate that human behaviour, perception, consciousness, environments and objects interlock to form a web of signs, psychoanalysts and others who work in the symbolic tradition have tended not to appreciate that signs are rooted in some environment, not a mentalistic netherworld. Rochberg-Halton attempts to resolve the tension between the environmentalist and semiological traditions by drawing on symbolic interactionist theory to develop a notion of 'cultivation' or the 'environmentally situated interpretive act'. His purpose in defining cultivation is to signify that 'the web of meaning that is the medium for the self is not merely a noun, "culture" . . . but is an active process of interpretation reciprocally requiring care and enquiry, and endowing one in turn with the broader perspective of community life'. He suggests that personal objects play an important role in this interpretative process because they 'act as signs of the self that are essential in their own right for its cultivation, and hence the world of meaning that we create for ourselves, and that creates ourselves, extends literally into the objective surroundings' (Rochberg-Halton 1984:344). To clarify this point, Rochberg-Halton is suggesting that personal objects are important mediators between self and the world. They serve as a display of personal meanings, but they also play a part in the psychosocial processes through which the self is constituted and maintained.

Rochberg-Halton's theory of cultivation is essentially a reformulation of one of the central arguments of Heidegger's *Being and Time*: that there is an interpretative dimension to human being. Chapter 7 showed that Heidegger's discussion of the role of interpretation in human life is his distinctive contribution to hermeneutical theory. Empirical support for the notion of cultivation is found in the work of Rubinstein (1989), who conducted a cultural-anthropological examination of the psychosocial processes linking person to place. His conclusions were developed during the course of hundreds of hours spent talking to older people in their homes. Rubinstein suggested that a 'person-centred process' constitutes one of the ways in which person and environment can be linked. Its four points offer a continuum on which the relationship of person and personal object can be plotted. These points are:

1 accounting;
2 personalisation;
3 extension;
4 embodiment.

They are discussed below.

## *Accounting*

The older person at home is intimately familiar with the configuration of the physical environment, and so can conduct everyday life with a minimum degree of difficulty. Rubinstein (1989) uses the term 'accounting' to describe this kind of knowledge of the environmental features of the home. He makes two observations:

1   Objects and environmental features vary with respect to their degree of significance: some things are rarely significant, while others are especially so.
2   There are at least two modes of significance. Some things, like tools, are significant because of what they enable their owners to do; while other things which are of little practical value are significant because they carry some special meaning.

Rubinstein found that, while it was comparatively rare for people to have an accurate mental inventory of all of the objects in the home environment, it was apparent that most objects had some kind of meaning, either as something merely owned or tolerated, or as occasionally useful, or in a more intimate way.

It follows, then, that significance is not so much an attribute or property of a thing in itself as a function of the relationship between that thing and its owner. Consequently, objects that are unrelated to current concerns tend to lose their significance and fade into the background. This is the meaning of Rubinstein's statement that 'accounting . . . incorporates the meaninglessness all environmental features have at times' (1989:48).

## Personalisation

Personalisation is the endowment of environmental features with meanings whose referents are the distinctive events, properties or projections of one's own life. It is the most modest level of involvement with environmental features.

## Extension

In 'extension', a greater degree of personal involvement with a feature occurs, and there is a more direct equation of the environmental feature with a part of the self. Individuals thus utilise environmental features as a direct and conscious representation of some key aspect of the self. This is illustrated by Sherman and Newman's (1977) study of the meanings of cherished possessions to a sample of ninety-four older people in community centres and nursing homes. A male respondent spoke of his violin, saying 'I am a musician, and the violin means everything to me' (p. 186). Referring to photographs of the family, a woman said 'They mean I was a woman. I had children and built my life around them. Happy memories' (p. 186). Equally, objects could be symbolic of important relationships. One woman said that her bracelet was her most cherished possession: 'My husband gave it to me sixty years ago. My feelings for him add much meaning to the object' (p. 186). These quotations amply demonstrate how personal possessions can act as 'signs of the self' (Rochberg-Halton 1984).

## *Embodiment*

Embodiment describes a relationship with objects or environmental features which have become so heavily charged with meaning as to be almost indistinguishable from the self. Rubinstein suggests that it can be important for older people who may feel that aspects of the environment have a greater potential for endurance than do their own bodies. He suggests that, through embodiment, environmental features may be assigned the task of carrying a load of personal meaning. In this way, they can aid in the maintenance of the self when it is threatened. Enlisted as an ally, an environmental feature can come to function as part prosthetic self.

The person-centred process is summarised in Box 9.1.

---

**Box 9.1 Summary of the person-centred process**

The four stages of the person-centred process differ with respect to the degree of interpenetration of person and environmental feature:

- Accounting is the base-line form.
- In personalisation, the hypothetical boundary between self and environment remains intact.
- In extension, it becomes blurred.
- In embodiment, it completely disappears.

In an earlier study, Rubinstein (1987) explored the meanings of personal objects to a sample of eighty-eight older people, who were asked to name and discuss the meaning of personally significant objects. Their responses were analytically sorted into a number of thematic categories, some of which add useful detail to the notion of the person-centred process.

## Connections with others

Rubinstein found that the largest category of meanings attributed to such objects involved connections with others, including grandparents, parents, children or spouses. Several subjects valued things that had been in the family for a number of generations, and were therefore symbolic of its continuity through time. Objects which had been handed on in this way helped their owners to see themselves as occupying important care-taking and custodial roles. An 84-year-old man spoke of his prized grandfather clock: 'It's been in the family for seven generations. It's gone to the eldest son in every generation.' At other times the value of objects was related to their status as gifts, either given or received. Older people who were moving into less spacious accommodation would sometimes give their property away to carefully chosen recipients; items which had been received as gifts gained value through their association with the giver.

## References to the self

A second large category of meanings related to objects which were important because they represented particular aspects of the self. Rubinstein describes the case of a woman who had built up a collection of 'old lady' dolls, each of which represented her at different periods in her old age; and that of an 87-year-old retired academic who continued to write scholarly works and who listed his typewriter, because it represented his continuing desire and ability to write. Respectively, these cases show the power of objects to represent the self as it is manifest in both being and doing.

## Defences against negative change

Another set of meanings for objects related to their properties as defences against change and negative events such as loss, boredom or loneliness. A 78-year-old woman valued her rocking chair, saying: 'I can't sit in it any more now that I broke my neck and I'm crippled, but I used to sit there in the evenings and talk to my husband when he was alive. Later, my children dubbed it "Granny's chair".' Objects were also valued as aids to overcoming boredom and loneliness. A 73-year-old woman listed her books: 'I read a lot. You can never be bored if you read.'

## Objects of care

A fourth group of meanings was related to objects which enabled their owners to express themselves through care. A woman mentioned her bird, her dog, and her plants, saying: 'These are things that need care, that need me. I have to be needed.'

## Objects of mature sensuousness

Rubinstein found that the significance of many objects had an affective or qualitative dimension, expressed in words such as 'liking', 'taste', 'comfort', 'warmth' and 'pride'. Beyond this, some objects appeared to be especially important because they embodied deeply held personal values and materially represented aspects of personal meaning systems.

## Objects as representations of the past

The final group of meanings was attached to objects significant as links to important events in the past, including childhood, married life, residence in another home, or the duration of the adult life.

Another study relevant here is described by Kalymun (1983), who interviewed elderly women about their decisions on retaining and disposing of personal possessions during relocation to new residential accommodation. Content analysis of interview transcriptions led to the development of a taxonomy of influencing factors. It was found that decisions were influenced both by environmental concerns, such as spatial features and the occasional existence of regulations, and by personal considerations. These included issues of function and utility, but once again the self-expressive role of personal objects was noted.

## The role of personal objects in the constitution of the home

In the light of the foregoing discussion, we can comment on the relationship between personal objects and the home. Rochberg-Halton (1984) notes that household artefacts do not exist atomistically, but form part of a *Gestalt* for the people who live with them. They communicate a sense of home, and also differentiate the types of activity that might be more appropriate for one part of the home than another. Thus, the meanings of a valued object are not limited to the thing itself, but also include its spatial context. In other words, one's personal possessions are not simply located in one's home, but help to constitute it as home. We therefore find that the interpretative process of cultivation Rochberg-Halton has described relates as much to the disposition and placement of artefacts as to the simple fact of their ownership. Rubinstein's work provides empirical justification for this suggestion. He argues that the decisions people make about room function, furniture placement and the use of decoration represent individual interpretations of sociocultural ideals. Rubinstein (1989) contends that culture suggests general rules for ordering and arranging space. The act of making order in a home, he argues, is a basic cultural act, and domestic order expresses basic cultural notions about personhood and social life. Simultaneously, the individual reproduces basic ideas about cultural order through the act of ordering the home, and interprets ideas about the cultural order. This process, which Rubinstein calls 'ordering', is another example of Rochberg-Halton's environmentally situated act of cultivation.

Personal objects play many important roles in the lives of older people. Those faced with change may use these objects in a manner analogous to the child's use of the transitional object, and may thereby find that they are better able to cope with the move from independent to institutional living (Sherman and Newman 1977). As noted above, these authors found a positive correlation between the ownership of a cherished personal possession and life satisfaction score; but beyond this, there is recurrent empirical and theoretical evidence for the proposition that personal objects support older people in their personhood. Goffman (1961) has noted that the personal possessions of an individual are an important part of the material out of which he or she builds a self, and Simone de Beauvoir has said that the older person's possessions assure him or her of his or her identity against those who claim to see him or her as nothing but an object (de Beauvoir 1973:699).

The ontological significance of personal objects has been explained by Rochberg-Halton's theory of cultivation, which argues that a person is related to the physical world through an active process of interpretation. According to this, personal objects are not simply a passive medium through which aspects of the self can be expressed; they also constitute key elements in a web of personal meanings, occasionally representing important aspects of the self, and playing a part in the psychosocial processes through which the self is constituted and maintained. In proposing a mechanism to show how personal meanings can extend into the objective surr-oundings of the physical world, the notion of cultivation offers a powerful theoretical perspective which helps us to understand the importance of home for older people.

## The importance of clothing

The role played by material artefacts in the interpretative processes of human being is illustrated with particular clarity by the case of clothing. The following extracts from the research text serve to illustrate its importance. The informant was talking about choice and control:

*Sister K*: I think the minute you walk through hospital doors that – that responsibility and control is taken away from you. Simply by taking off your clothes and putting you in pyjamas or a white gown in casualty. You strip them of their identity in a way, by putting a white gown on.

*Researcher*: So there is more in taking somebody's clothes away than just removing what they're wearing?
*Sister K*: Yes.

Later, Sister K described her personal experience of the loss of control involved in wearing a white gown.

*Sister K*: I think it's foul. I've only ever once had a medical examination, and it was the most embarrassing thing that I've ever been through. It was the time when I felt least in control.
*Researcher*: Yes.
*Sister K*: Because I felt not only that I was physically naked, but I felt mentally naked as well.
*Researcher*: Mentally naked?
*Sister K*: It was a terrible feeling.
*Researcher*: What do you mean by mentally naked?
*Sister K*: I felt so vulnerable.

This informant's perception of a link between personal identity and clothing is justified by the research-based literature. Veblen (1953) was one of the earliest writers to argue that clothing did more than protect the body. Rudd (1992) argued that clothing is a rich example of a cultural sign system which has strong communicative value and is used by individuals, groups and cultures to negotiate meaning and interact on the basis of that meaning. Kaiser (1990) drew upon semiotics and social psychology to propose a model linking the structural analysis of appearance with the social processes engaged through appearance in constructing meaning.

The anthropologists Roach and Bubolz-Eicher (1979) argue that the human practices of personal adornment and dressing are communicative acts that serve critical functions in human societies. They claim that these practices support the individual in his or her endeavour to appear as a unique person and provide a way of expressing, reinforcing, initiating or camouflaging mood. These researchers also identify a number of socially useful functions fulfilled by clothing, shown in Box 9.2.

Social psychologists have examined the role played by clothing in the presentation of self, and person perception (Davis and Lennon

**Box 9.2 Social functions of clothing**

- identifying social worth;
- symbolising economic status;
- representing political power or ideological orientation;
- reflecting magico-religious condition;
- reinforcing beliefs, customs and values.

1988). Eriksen and Sirgy (1992) found that employed women were more likely to wear outfits at work that matched their actual and ideal self images; Kwon and Farber (1992) reported that the style of dress often affects the perception of the wearer's professionalism, intelligence and competence; and Rudd (1992) described the sign value of the dress patterns of a group of homosexual men.

Cordwell and Schwarz (1979) offer an assessment of the role of clothing that is fully congruent with Heidegger's notion of interpretation and Rochberg-Halton's concept of cultivation. The latter suggests that clothing helps to define a person's relationship with the sociocultural and the natural environments, and that the study of clothing and adornment is significant as an anthropological enterprise. For Cordwell and Schwarz, the significance of clothing lies in the symbolic role that it plays in mediating the relationship between nature, the individual and the sociocultural environment.

The relationship of clothing to quality of life is discussed in more detail in the next chapter.

## Summary

This chapter has discussed places, personal possessions and clothing in terms of the meanings they have for older people. The concepts of being-in-the-world and interpretation have offered a theoretical perspective from which to address the text, and evidence from the empirical literature has been introduced to enrich and corroborate the findings. The content of this chapter has important implications for the nursing care of the older person in the hospital or nursing home environment.

We have noted that the importance of personal possessions is not limited to their practical function as tools that help us in our daily lives, but that they also play important symbolic roles of various kinds and are intimately related to the ways in which we regard ourselves and other people. It is interesting to reflect that the rituals of admission to hospital often involve taking off one's normal, everyday clothing, and replacing it with the uniform of 'the patient', which normally takes the form of night-clothes or some sort of white gown. Wearing the uniform of a patient often involves a lack of dignity. Hospital night-clothes and gowns rarely fit well, and one is constantly aware that certain body parts may be more visible to the public gaze than is normally the case. It should now be clear that a second and more fundamental indignity occurs, associated with a change in social status from that of autonomous individual to that of hospital patient.

This change in status has a number of functions. One of these may be to make it less embarrassing and difficult for nursing staff to offer intimate personal care. We should also remember that the change in status from autonomous individual to hospital patient is often accompanied by loss of personal power and increased vulnerability.

# Chapter 10
# Being an individual

When they were asked to discuss quality of life, many people used the word 'individual': quality of life was seen to be an individual thing, individuality was a property that must be respected, and quality of life depended upon individualised care. The tendency to link individuality and quality of life is illustrated in the following extract from the text:

*Sister O*: Treating people as individuals increases the quality of their lives. Not treating them as individuals and telling them what is happening is detrimental to their quality of life.

Although many members of staff who were interviewed identified a link between quality of life and being treated as an individual, most were unable to go beyond a simple statement to justification of their position. For instance, when Sister P was asked why we should treat people as individuals, she said that it was because they *were* individuals. Sister N also suggested that people should be treated as individuals because they are individuals, and she found it difficult to go beyond this point.

All references to the individual in the research data imply that it is a goal to be aimed at, a state to be approved of, or a generally 'good thing': no one said that to be or to be treated as an individual was undesirable. However, asked why being an individual was such a good thing, people were unable to say. For most of the people interviewed, then, the state of being an individual was regarded as a fact that is self-evidently true, and a goal that is evidently desirable. As individuality is a widely held and largely unexamined assumption that underpins the thinking of many of the carers who were interviewed, it can be described as a principle or axiom.

## The nature of individuality: an historical perspective

Historically, the notion of individualism has carried widely varying connotations. One of the earliest references to the individual is found in the Bible, where, in the book of Ezekiel, the prophet rejects the earlier teaching that children should pay the penalty for the sins of their fathers, and argues that people should bear responsibility for the outcome of their own actions. Elsewhere in the Bible the notion of individualism denotes that national and social categories are of little significance to God: 'there is neither Greek nor Jew, circumcision nor uncircumcision, Barbarian, Scythian, bond nor free: but Christ is all, and in all' (Colossians 3:2).

Lukes (1973) has written a history of the development of the idea of individualism in Europe and America from 1820 to 1974. He claims that the concept expresses five basic ideas, shown in Box 10.1.

---

**Box 10.1  Key ideas of individualism**

- The *dignity of the individual* expresses the 'ultimate moral principle of the supreme and intrinsic value, or dignity, of the individual human being' (Lukes 1973:45). This ideal received systematic expression in the work of Kant, who asserted that people exist as ends in themselves, and not merely as a means for arbitrary use by others.
- *Autonomy* is the idea that every person has the ability and the right to think and to make judgements and decisions for himself or herself.
- *Privacy* describes a private domain in which the individual has the right to do whatever he or she chooses.
- The principle of *self-development* promotes the complete realisation of an individual's unique potential.
- The *abstract individual* is a way of conceptualising the individual in terms of needs, interests, wants or other purposes that are assumed to be common to all people, irrespective of specific social and historical circumstances.

Lukes argues that these five basic ideas of individualism have given rise to six doctrines of individualism (summarised here as by Wilkie 1986):

1 Economic individualism is the doctrine of *laissez-faire* capitalism, including the principle of free trade.
2 Political individualism is the core principle of representative democracy, as expressed in the slogan 'one person one vote'.
3 Religious individualism refers to the doctrines of individual salvation and conscience.
4 Ethical individualism expresses the same doctrine in a secular form.
5 Methodological individualism is the idea that all valid explanations of social phenomena can be reduced to the thoughts, feelings and motives of individuals.
6 Epistemological individualism is the doctrine that the sources and criteria of valid knowledge are individual, not social.

The principle of individualism has often been invoked in political debate. In England, the philosopher John Stuart Mill (1879) decried a contemporary political system based on individualism as vicious and antisocial. He described socialism as a system in which each person was for herself or himself and against all the rest; which was grounded in the opposition of interests instead of harmony; and under which everyone was required to find her or his place by a struggle, by pushing others back, or being pushed back by them. Mill considered such a system to be economically and morally fatal.

The principle of individualism seems to have been received more positively in the United States of America at the turn of the present century. There, according to Lukes (1973), it was regarded as the actual or imminent realisation of the final stage of human progress in a spontaneously cohesive society of equal individual rights, limited government, *laissez-faire*, natural justice and equal opportunity.

In contemporary Britain, the notion of the individual is often invoked in the context of a political debate about the respective roles of the individual and society (see for instance Thatcher 1993). The tension between the individual and social poles of human life is not unique to politics, but can also be found in the philosophical literature and the research text (see below).

## Promoting individuality

Nursing staff interviewed during this research recognised the individuality of older people by acknowledging that they differ in respect of their aims, goals and expectations. The terms 'purpose' and 'aim' were used both in a global and in a more limited sense. Used globally, they can refer to a person's purpose in life:

*Sister Q*: I don't know really – I don't know if it is something we give enough thought to really, what's their purpose in life? I mean, we know what our purpose is for them, but actually thinking about what their purpose is, I'm not sure.

*Researcher*: One of the sisters said she never used to ask things like that because she was frightened they might turn around and say, 'I haven't got a purpose in life.'

*Sister Q*: I think you might get that answer here: 'My purpose is to die.'

The following quotation refers to 'purpose' in a more limited sense:

*Sister N*: You've got to include things like good health, really, basic needs being met like shelter, food, emotional needs being met as well, like being loved, being cared for, being wanted, things like that really, and perhaps some sort of purpose in life as well you know, like people have a job or a hobby, something that's important to them.

Thus, it appears that there are shades of meaning to 'purpose', ranging from short-term objectives, through pastimes, hobbies, occupations and jobs, to a broad goal towards which the whole of one's life is oriented.

If we move beyond attitudes to behaviour, it appears that treating people as individuals first involves a demonstration of respect for their purposes:

*Sister L*: A difficult question, and without going away and thinking about it, off the top of my head, treating them like an individual, not like children, like an individual and have time to sit and listen to what they want, what are their expectations, what do they want out of life. Let's face it, the majority that come here only have five years to live, and I don't think we should make any hard and fast rules. I think it's important to sit down and think about what are their expectations, what would they like to do, what they want to achieve.

Having recognised the existence of individual purposes, it is then necessary to enable the person to express them:

*Researcher*: How exactly do you treat them as individuals? What is important?
*Charge Nurse S*: We try to take into account all their preference, as far as you can with a ward routine – as far as is possible to take into account all their individual preferences for dressing, washing and so on.

The interview transcriptions show that in practice, the recognition and expression of individual preferences often involve the issues of choice and control, and these issues will now be discussed.

## Individuality, choice and control

The related issues of choice and control appear throughout the data. Sister K felt that freedom of choice in decision making was important because it characterised self-responsibility and gave individuals control over their own lives. Further probing exposed her assumption that self-responsibility, self-control and expression of the self through choice were self-evidently good. The axiomatic nature of self-determination was also demonstrated by Sister P, who felt that treating people as individuals was an important way of promoting quality of life. When asked to justify this statement, she argued that people must be treated as individuals because 'that is what they are', and echoed the sentiments of the many informants whose opening remarks at interview were that the 'quality of life is an individual thing'. Sister T went a step further, suggesting that freedom of choice and the right to self-determination were defining characteristics of humanity and gifts from God:

*Sister N*: I think the most important word I would suggest is an element of choice . . . Choice has got to be the most important thing, I'd say.

The range of issues over which choices could be made was enumerated several times:

*Sister K*: Everything from when you have a meal, to when you have a wash, to when you get up on a morning, to whether you decide to take some medical advice or not . . . or where you're going to live, everything. From getting up on a morning, to deciding whether you're going to move from your home into an old people's home.

And:

*Sister T*: Choice in where they sit to eat their meals, choice in what time they get up and go to bed, choice in what they eat. Then similar to choice is control – that they should have some control over what's done with them, particularly in hospital, that they're given some control over what treatment they have.

Some informants were asked to explain why choice was such an important issue in quality of life:

*Sister T*: I think because of the way it's linked with control. If we have choice we have control over ourselves. And if control over ourselves is removed, then you don't feel you're a person. You're dehumanised, somehow.
*Researcher*: So is there some kind of link between quality of life and being a person?
*Sister T*: Well you can make them less of a person by taking away their control and choice. I think they're then less of a person.

Sister T asserts that choice and control have ontological significance. This view is confirmed by Macquarrie (1972), who argues that what is really chosen is the self. Following Heidegger, he suggests that the self is not ready-made at the beginning of life. What is given, he suggests, is a 'field of possibility'. As people '[project themselves] into this possibility rather than that one', so they begin to determine who they will be.

It is relatively easy to see that major life choices such as one's career path or the decision to parent shape the emerging self, but the data suggest that everyday choices can also have ontological significance. An extract from the interview with Sister K offers a concrete example. It concerns choice of clothing, a material artefact whose symbolic significance was indicated in Chapter 9.

*Researcher*: So somehow it seems as if you are saying that an important part of quality of life is having choice.
*Sister K*: Yes.
*Researcher*: And one of the things we make choices about is how we dress. Because I suppose that's how we express ourselves?
*Sister K*: That's me. I dress quite loudly. I like to dress quite brightly because that's part of my personality, and I'm sure it's the same with everybody else.

If, as this informant argues, clothing is important as a sign of the self, it may follow that decisions about dress may have deeper implications:

*Researcher*: And when people come into hospital and we take their clothes off them, we take more than their clothes off?
*Sister K*: Yes.
*Researcher*: I'm just checking that I've got your story right.
*Sister K*: Yes. We take more than their clothes. I think so anyway.
*Researcher*: We take their choice away from them.
*Sister K:* Yes. And we take responsibility away from them.
*Researcher*: Responsibility for what?
*Sister K:* Perhaps responsibility is not the right word. By taking their clothes off them you make them vulnerable, so they become dependent on us.
*Researcher*: Right.
*Sister K:* And because they're so dependent on us we take responsibility as well. That's what I mean.

Sister R also understood that clothing was an important marker of human being. She had developed a system where patients could have name-tags put into their clothes within an hour of their arrival in hospital, in order to prevent institutional clothing being worn or a night spent in hospital pyjamas.

Other members of staff were also concerned with the practicalities of providing choice. At the simplest level, it was recognised that time is an important raw material if choice is to be provided:

*Sister Q* (describing personalised clothing): You need to have someone to put them away, and you can have five or six bags of
clothing waiting to be sorted and put into the ward, and you
think, well you just can't do it, so you resort to ward stock, and
you might have six bags there full of clothes for this person and
you can't find any. So you need to have somebody to do that.

Time was also regarded as an important prerequisite to the development of the kind of relationship in which people could most
easily be treated as individuals. In an unrecorded interview, Sister Y
said that the most important component of care was sitting down
and chatting with patients, as it allowed you to get to know them as
people as well as patients. This kind of relationship was also promoted when care was organised appropriately. It seems that the
staff seem most able to treat people as individuals when this is
done so that a nurse has responsibility for a particular group of
patients over a period of time:

*Sister Q*: We try to treat everybody . . . we work very much in
groups on the ward, so we've got four groups of mixed ability
patients, and one nurse is allocated to that group in the morning.
So she knows who she's looking after, there are her patients, and
it's for her to ensure that the care is given. I think that helps a
little.

The organisation of care will be discussed in more detail in the
next chapter.

It has been shown that the text links quality of life of the older
person to control and the exercise of choice. Empirical literature
relating to this issue will now be discussed.

## Control and the well-being of the older person

In psychology, control has been defined as the individual's perception that he or she can execute (or has the potential to execute)
some action that changes an aversive stimulus (Miller and Combs
1989). Early experimental studies into control conducted by psychologists in the 1960s and 1970s are reviewed in Averill (1973),
Miller (1979) and Thompson (1981). These reviews conclude that

reactions to the presence or absence of control are not easy to predict because they depend on the meaning of the situation to the individual (Averill 1973). Folkman (1984) proposes that the meaning of a situation is determined by a two-stage process of appraisal:

1  In primary appraisal, the person judges whether the event is a threat to her or his well-being. This judgement is influenced by the controllability of the situation and the person's belief in her or his ability to influence outcomes (locus of control).
2  Secondary appraisal involves assessment of the available options and coping responses in each specific situation. This is influenced by individual coping strategies and self-efficacy beliefs (Bandura 1977).

Individuals' perceptions of control can influence their health (Langer 1983, Moore and Schulz 1987), self-esteem (Langer 1983, Moore and Schulz 1987), anxiety (Lefcourt 1982), depression (Langer 1983, Moore and Schulz 1987), activity (Arling *et al.* 1986), and life satisfaction (Arling *et al.* 1986, Moore and Schulz 1987).

The construct of control is highly relevant to this discussion, because there is evidence that institutional regimes of the type found in some nursing homes are likely to lessen residents' actual (Storlie 1982) or perceived control over their environment (Gifford 1987, Langer 1983, Palmore *et al.* 1985). A range of studies has shown that perceived loss of control is associated with deterioration in the health and well-being of older people. Wolk and Telleen (1976) found that satisfaction and developmental task accomplishment of a group of 129 elderly people were inversely related to the perceived level of constraint of the residential setting.

Langer and Rodin (1976) conducted a field experiment to assess the effect of control on a range of actions designed to improve the well-being of older people in nursing homes. Residents allocated to the experimental group were given a communication emphasising their responsibility for themselves, whereas those in the control group were given a communication stressing the staff's responsibility for them. In addition, the former group was given the freedom to make choices and the responsibility of caring for a plant rather than having decisions made and the plant taken care of for them by the staff. Rodin and Langer report that measures of alertness, active participation and general sense of well-being showed a significant improvement for the experimental group. Rodin and Langer (1979) reported that the beneficial effects were still visible eighteen months later, and even that the death rate was reduced in the experimental group.

The work of Rodin and Langer contains certain methodological flaws that limit confidence in their findings. They failed to demonstrate that members of the experimental and control groups were equivalent in respect of their locus of control. Cicirelli (1987) later reported that people with an external locus of control were better adjusted to institutional life, and Hickson *et al.* (1988) and Mancini (1987) reported a significant association between higher life satisfaction and internal locus of control. Rodin and Langer's control and experimental groups were also on separate floors of the building. The researchers acknowledge that there was little communication between floors, and it is possible, for we are not told otherwise, that each was serviced by its own team of nurses. Subsequent nursing research (Baker 1978) has demonstrated that the well-being of resident patients can be influenced by the leadership style of senior nurses, and the presence of a dynamic nurse leader on the experimental floor could easily explain the perceived effect.

More recent studies into the effect of control-relevant interventions, conducted under tighter control, have supported some of Rodin and Langer's findings. Banziger and Roush (1983) randomly allocated nursing home residents to one of three groups:

1   The control-relevant group received a message invoking responsibility and were given the chance to care for a bird-table.
2   The dependency group were given a message invoking dependency and were not given the opportunity to care for a bird-table.
3   This group received neither intervention.

The researchers found that the control-relevant group scored more highly on a measure of life satisfaction, while there was no difference between the scores of the other two groups. Finally,

Chowdhary (1990) found that the sense of control and the self-esteem of institutionalised older men were enhanced when they were given control over the choice of clothing to wear.

## The limits of individuality

Although it appears that promoting individuality through the provision of choice is regarded by the staff as self-evidently desirable, they recognise that under a range of circumstances the choices offered to older people in hospital care might be severely limited. Hence the note of caution in the following extract:

*Sister N*: Choice has got to be the most important thing, I'd say, that people can choose to some extent . . . as far as is possible, I do believe that people should have a choice.

The limits to choice will now be discussed. It will first be shown that the staff believe aspects of the organisational structure can limit the choices available to older people; second, a range of deliberate strategies used by the staff themselves to limit choice will be described; and third, the ways in which they justify the use of these strategies will be explored. Finally, the tension between forces that tend to promote individuality, and those that tend to suppress it, will be placed in the context of hermeneutical theory.

## *Limiting choice*

Ward sisters identified certain aspects of the organisational structure as limiting factors in the provision of choice. Commonly, it was argued that understaffing or shortage of time restricted care to the provision of the basics. Sister K spelt out resource problems in some detail.

*Sister K*: . . . lack of physical resources . . . you have the expertise to prevent someone from developing an uncomfortable pressure sore, but you don't have the equipment, thus the development of the pressure sore will reduce their quality of life. If you don't have enough staff, if you only have enough to rush around everywhere, and make sure everyone is clean and dressed or being fed, and not enough time to have any social talk or negotiations, then that prevents you from giving them quality of life. And then there's the expertise of the staff. If they don't have the . . . professional knowledge base they won't know what's the right thing to do and to treat. And if they don't have the skills in terms of interpersonal skills, they won't be able to enhance people's choice and help them to feel encouraged or motivated . . . so I think resources on all these levels have a great input.

Choice could also be restricted by health authority policy such as restriction of smoking facilities (Sister N). The text expresses doubt as to whether restrictions of this kind work for the long-term benefit of the patient. This is illustrated through reference to health education:

*Sister K*: I think the key is helping people to help themselves to do the things they want to do when they want to do them. It's difficult because there are some circumstances, like health education really, that's contrary to that. But it's difficult to promote health education . . . if it's not going to satisfy someone. I just think about myself . . . if someone said to me 'You must lose three stone', it would absolutely devastate me, because part of my quality of life is being able to eat what I want when I want, and to enjoy it. Like elderly men who smoke a lot, and doctors say 'Stop smoking', but that's an enjoyment and a pleasure to them. I just think as long as they have the two sets of facts in front of them, then that's their decision.

Sometimes, people forego their choices to please other people. Sister O described the case of an elderly woman who had requested a side-room because she enjoyed the solitude and was able to read there in peace. However, her husband was upset by her apparent isolation, and so she spent more and more time in the communal areas of the ward 'to stop the nurses getting into trouble' and to please her husband. This illustrates the way freedom of choice is limited by situational factors (Benner and Wrubel 1989).

There were several other ways in which choice could be restricted. As Sister N commented, some patients were too ill to recognise the alternatives available to them, and therefore to choose. Sister P discriminated between the provision of choice and its exercise, suggesting that patients should always be offered a choice as 'just to do things for them could be degrading'. As we have seen, the psychological literature defines control as the individual's perception that he or she can bring about change. Where older people are genuinely unable to make a choice, for whatever reason, then the provision of information can also ameliorate the stressful consequences of loss of control, to some degree (Johnson 1975, Wilson-Barnett 1980).

There were circumstances in which sisters felt themselves justified in deliberately restricting the choices they offered to patients in particular phases of illness. Elderly people sometimes select a course of action felt to be inappropriate or unwise by the staff involved in their care. This causes the potential for conflict. The kinds of circumstance where this might happen were described by Sister U:

*Sister U*: It's very difficult because a lot of the elderly live on their own . . . sometimes they don't want anyone intruding into their home. It can be quite a problem because we've had a lot of elderly that don't want home helps going in because they don't want them to know what's in the house, they don't want them to see their pension book. It's very difficult because you're taking that patient's independence away.

The nature of the conflict in these cases was nicely summarised by Sister T:

*Sister T*: Most things are achievable. Where it becomes more difficult is where I feel a certain course of action would be therapeutic and important for their treatment and they don't.

In such cases, one logical possibility is that the staff will concede any choice made by patients. The text does not suggest that any of the staff advocated or practised such an approach: all who discussed this issue seemed to accept that there were circumstances in which it was legitimate to override or modify the wishes of the patient. A range of different mechanisms might be employed.

## *Deliberate strategies*

### Coming to a compromise

Coming to a compromise is a mechanism whereby the nurse restricts the choices available to the patient to a number of options from which he or she may choose. Sister T described this approach in the context of rehabilitation:

*Sister T*: It might be that you come to a compromise with the patient whereby they walk to one end of their bed and get the wheelchair there. And so though you've said to their initial response that they couldn't walk at all, 'No, that isn't an option', then you've given them an option of what distance they do walk; or you might say you've got to walk one way, and do they want to walk to lunch, or would they rather wait and walk back? But whatever, you can still provide options, so you can still provide choices, but you're limiting it. I think that's a more constructive way forward.

### Massive encouragement

There were circumstances in which the staff felt justified in compelling a patient to do certain things. Sister T, once again, describes circumstances in which she might take this action:

*Sister T*: In situations of acute illness, and at the beginning of rehabilitation when it is such an effort for somebody they don't want to try. For example with walking, they want you to wheel them because they can't possibly walk, and yet once you've been teaching them to walk, and making them walk increasingly by stages you eventually find that they are not only able to walk but can do it by themselves. And then that gives them more choice because then they can choose when to get up and where to go.

The sisters felt justified in restricting the choices available to such patients by compelling them to walk to the toilet, but then pushing them back in a wheelchair. Sister P called this 'massive encouragement', and believed it was valid if it resulted in such an improvement in the patients' condition that eventually their range of options was enlarged. If on the other hand a patient was terminally ill or no improvement could realistically be anticipated, no such restriction on choice would be imposed.

### Forcing and physical restraint

Despite the emphasis nursing staff placed on the principle of individuality and freedom of choice, there were circumstances in which some nurses were prepared to impose their own aims and goals and to over-ride those of the patient completely:

*Researcher*: Do you think that there are circumstances where we are right to take decisions for the patient, to take away their choice?

*Sister Q*: Yes, I'm sure we do all the time anyway. It's like putting a patient into a Buxton chair. We've got a man who wanders around. That's OK. He lies on the floor. That's no problem because we've not got many who walk, but it gets to a point where he's rushing around and he's likely to either fall and knock himself or knock something over and hurt somebody else. So at that time we say right, OK, he's got to go into a chair, so we are really restricting him in a way, restraining him. I don't like the word restrain, but we're protecting him, protecting other people, so we put him in a chair.

In the most extreme case, nurses were prepared to use physical force in order to impose their will upon that of the patient:

*Sister Q*: This man we're talking about, he's had a stroke so all down his left side he's got no movement at all. Now ideally, you should approach him from his left side. You approach him from this side he's not going to hit you, and see if you can get it done . . . and try to get it done as quickly as possible, really. The more you try to communicate with him the more he's hitting you, and there comes a time when you think, 'Let's get on with it, stop him doing this', and we do it pretty quickly and ask for help, two of us to do him.

Such strategies have a degree of success in an institutional setting only. Sister R, a district nurse, was asked what would happen if attempts were made to force people in their own homes. She felt that forcing did not happen as much in the community. She acknowledged that patients might perhaps do as they are told in the presence of the nurse, but denied that this would have any lasting effect on their behaviour. She felt there was little use in trying to force compliance, and that it was much more productive to try to enlist patients' co-operation.

Sister V, another district nurse, similarly said that forcing 'just could not be done' in the community, as patients would tell you to leave.

### Controlling information

Limiting the older person's ability to choose can happen covertly, as well as overtly. Sister K argued that providing or retaining information could be a subtle way of shaping the choices made by patients:

*Sister K*: I think we play at informed choice. We pretend that we do it. We pretend that we give adequate information and enable patients to make a choice, but I don't think we do really. I think we just give them what we want them to know. Generally, nurses are extremely bad at communicating and laying unbiased both sides of the story, putting information at the patient's disposal.

Other aspects of the data also show that nurses are selective in the information that they pass on to patients. Although, for instance, Social Worker W felt that it was right in principle to give patients full and complete information, he accepted that there were cases where this might not be desirable in practice. The decision about how much information would be given was taken in the context of the nurse's relationship with the patient, often after assessing his or her capacity to understand, or 'how much he or she wanted to know':

*Sister M*: Yes, within their capabilities I don't think you should upset patients with unnecessary information, and there is a lot of unnecessary information when you are talking about prognosis and diagnosis – 'Well it might be this', or 'We ought to check that' – before you really know, and I think you've got to be careful, you know: 'We are doing tests to see what might be wrong' is better than 'We think it might be such and such', which is unnecessary chitter for the patient.

Sister Q worked on a ward which served as a final home for many of its residents. This was one thing she did not want her patients to know:

*Researcher*: So everybody here has accepted that this is the end of the line, really?
*Sister Q*: Yes.
*Researcher*: Do you think the patients know?
*Sister Q*: I don't know. I'd like to think no, they don't.
*Researcher*: Why?
*Sister Q*: Because I'd hate to think it was like a death sentence.
*Research Assistant*: A dumping ground?
*Sister Q*: Yes. It's been said it's the last step, and the only way you'll get out is in a box, stuff like that. And, while looking after somebody who's dying is important, looking after them while they are living is more important really.
*Researcher*: You said sometimes you don't want them to know as it would be like a death sentence, so you don't really believe in some cases . . .?
*Sister Q*: No, what I mean is, if somebody is dying, elderly, frail and dying, well yes you are, are you comfortable is the issue. What I mean by that is I'd hate somebody to think I'm going into [names ward] tomorrow to die. You might say yes you will, but it might be this year, or next, or five years' time. So while it's part of what we do, it's only a little part. I'd hate to think they think it's a death sentence coming here, but yes, realistically it's the last stop.

## *The paradox of individuality*

This analysis of the principle of individuality reveals a clear tension between the expressed beliefs and the actions of caring staff. On the one hand, hospital staff have strongly endorsed the promotion of individuality by facilitating patient choice; on the other, they describe a range of mechanisms through which older people are effectively denied the opportunity to make choices. This conflict might be called 'the paradox of individuality'. The interviews show that many of the staff were aware of this paradox and sought to justify or explain it, often on altruistic grounds. In the following case, Sister Q was defending her use of the Buxton chair:

*Researcher*: So it's like physical danger, really?

*Sister Q*: Yes. It's when we feel he's going to be a danger to himself or others. So he's in a chair now. He might not like being in a chair, but we feel he's safer like that. But whether it's right . . . I think we're always going to be doing that, and I think as long as you can say it's in the patient's best interests, then for me it's OK. As long as it's not in the nurse's best interest, as long as it's for the patient, then that's it. There are patients who are in Buxton chairs, and it's not on here, well I hope not on here, at least not when I'm on, and it's often for the nurses. So I think that's wrong.

In the quotation given earlier, this informant took care to redefine restraint as protection. She seems unsure whether it is a proper course of action ('but whether it's right . . .'). Finally, she is at pains to distance herself from the use of Buxton chairs, claiming that they are not used on her ward but another, and even if they are used on her ward it is not when she is there, and then always for the benefit of the patient (although on wards other than hers it might be for the benefit of the staff). It may be that this distancing of self from an action that self has undertaken results from conflict arising from espousing the principle of individuality, and acting in ways which effectively deny choice; but ultimately, the informant justifies the occasional use of restraint in the Buxton chair on the grounds of altruism, or being 'in the patient's best interests'. Other members of staff argued in the same way. A physiotherapist claimed that her goal was to make patients 'carry on and be as independent as possible'. She felt that those who did not want to be independent were 'lazy' or had a 'mental problem'. In the long term, forcing patients was for their own good.

### Limiting choice and the ethos of expertise

We have seen that the individuality of the older person in hospital can be impaired by the controlling activities of the nursing staff, through mechanisms such as massive encouragement and forcing. The paradox of individuality is that the staff who employ these controlling mechanisms are often enthusiastic advocates of the individuality of the older person. It has been shown that staff sometimes attempt to resolve or explain this paradox by claiming that their actions are taken for the greater good of the patient. Sister K offered a rather different analysis, arguing that the restriction of patient choice was a routine affair that had little to do with altruism. She claimed that control and choice were often taken away from people as soon as they are admitted to hospital, giving the examples of clothing (quoted in Chapter 9) and medication:

*Sister K*: I think medication is about the clearest example.

*Researcher*: Right.

*Sister K*: We automatically assume it's best for that patient, as soon as they get through the doors, to take their tablets off them, and start giving them out of the trolley . . . and that's a big responsibility taken away from the patient.

This informant argues that nurses assume responsibility for their patients because nurses have an ethos of expertise which is strengthened through association with the medical profession. One consequence is that autonomous and questioning patients are found to be threatening:

*Sister K*: I think we feel that people – we're the experts and we know best. And if they [the patients] say 'Well, I don't want to do that, and I don't think you know best', then that's quite threatening.

*Researcher*: It's a threat to our professional ego?

*Sister K*: Yes, yes.

*Researcher*: Lots of times people have come into hospital and said, 'I want to die'; and we don't respect that choice.

*Sister K:* We think that they must be wrong.

*Researcher*: Yes, we say they must be depressed.

*Sister K*: And doctors won't accept that. Doctors find that really very difficult to accept, that somebody makes that choice. It's like going against their Hippocratic Oath, or whatever, and because we're still a sort of semi-extension of them we don't help. We don't help to put the patient's point of view.

The quotation links the paradox of individualism to carers' professional belief systems, and thus to the wider social context in which care is practised. Sister K felt that it was not simply the actions of individual members of staff, but the social structure of the hospital itself, that constrained the exercise of choice by patients:

*Researcher*: The institution has a particular goal, and the goal is that you will come in here, and you will get healthy, and you will go out again?

*Sister K*: Yes. You will do it as quickly as possible, and with the least possible problems, and the least difficulty, and you've got to be . . . got to be a happy patient that doesn't ask questions, and you can't be incontinent, and you can't be difficult.

At the heart of Sister K's analysis is her perception that the personal goals of the older person in hospital may conflict with medically defined priorities. She implies that the real purpose of the controlling strategies (negotiating, forcing, etc.) is to shape the goals of the older person to those of 'the system'; or failing this, to override them. She argues that this process begins during admission to hospital, through mechanisms that accomplish and signify the change in status from independent person to hospital patient. These may include dressing the person in night-wear, and controlling her or his access to medication. The person who conforms to medical priorities and goals may come to be regarded as a 'model patient', although the cost of this achievement is increased vulnerability and surrendered autonomy. People who are reluctant to subscribe to the goals of the hospital may occupy the alternative role of 'difficult patient':

*Sister K*: The problem I have on the ward when they're difficult patients is when they feel they're out of control. That's when you have most problems, when they feel that they haven't got any responsibility and haven't got any control. And we label them 'difficult patients'.

There will be further discussion of the relationship between the organisation of care and the quality of life of the older person in the next chapter.

# Perspectives on the principle of individuality

Aspects of Heidegger's work usefully inform the foregoing discussion. First, the relationship will be explored between the principle of individuality and the Heideggerian concept of existence. As we have seen in Chapter 7, this concept is central to Heidegger's work. Cooper (1992) suggests that no complete account can be given of a human being without reference to what he or she is in the process of becoming and to the projects and intentions which he or she is on the way to realising, and in terms of which sense is made of his or her present condition.

The principle of individuality, as it is found in the interview transcriptions, is congruent with this concept of existence. The data assert that the individuality of older people is recognised as their differing goals and expectations are acknowledged, and that their individuality is promoted as the staff preserve and enhance their ability to make choices about their lives.

It is clear too that staff attitudes, and actions such as physical restraint, information restriction and forcing, neither acknowledge nor promote the individuality of the older person in hospital care. The hermeneutical tradition also provides an interesting perspective on this feature.

We have seen that for Heidegger, human being is being-in-the-world: that the physical world is saturated with meaning, and that the relationship between the human being and that world is one of necessary interdependence. He also recognises, however, that there is a social dimension to human being: for existentialists such as Heidegger, individuality and sociality constitute inescapable poles of human life. Cooper (1992) notes that the person is, on the one hand, a free, meaning-giving, existing individual and, on the other hand, a necessary participant in a public, social world. Between these poles, it is possible for the individual to live either an authentic or an inauthentic life, as outlined in Box 10.2.

The complementary notions of authentic and inauthentic being-with-others enable us to evaluate the various ways the staff justify the limitations they place on the older person's ability to choose. Although techniques such as massive encouragement (see pp. 134–5) place temporary restriction on the older person's facility

### Box 10.2 Authentic and inauthentic lives

Cooper (1992) explains that the word 'authentic' reflects the meaning of the Greek word from which it derives, which means 'a person who does things for himself or herself'. In the German, this word is translated as '*eigen*', which means 'own', as in 'ownership'.

Macquarrie (1972) considers the criteria by which we can distinguish between authentic and inauthentic being-with-others. He suggests that authentic being-with-others is the mode of relation to the other that promotes existence in the full sense by letting the human stand out as human, in freedom and responsibility. Inauthentic being-with-others, on the other hand, suppresses the genuinely human and personal.

For Macquarrie, whatever kind of relation to others depersonalises and dehumanises is an inauthentic one. He recognises a paradox: a purely individual existence is not possible and could not properly be called an 'existence'; yet existence with others is authentic to the degree that it lets individuals be free to become the unique persons that they are. For Macquarrie, true community allows for true diversity.

of self-determination, they are sometimes justified by staff on the grounds that they enhance the range of options available to that older person in the future. Other techniques, such as forcing and physical restraint, even though they may be justified in altruistic terms, do nothing to promote the future independence of the person, but probably make life a little easier for the staff. These two approaches correspond with Heidegger's description of two forms of solicitude:

1  'that which leaps in and dominates';
2  'that which leaps forth and liberates'.

The former, inauthentic form of solicitude 'takes over for the other that with which he is to concern himself'. The other, in Heidegger's words, is thrown out of his position; he 'steps back, so that after-wards, when the matter has been attended to, he can either take it over as something finished and at his disposal, or disburden himself of it completely'. The alternative, authentic form of solicitude 'leaps ahead' of the other, 'not in order to take away his care but to give it back to him authentically as such for the first time . . . it helps the other to become transparent to himself in his career and to become free for it' (Heidegger 1962:158).

## Summary

This chapter has explored various aspects of the principle of individuality. It has been shown that members of staff claim individuality is an important characteristic of older people, although they are rarely able to justify this opinion explicitly. Various approaches to promoting individuality have been discussed as they were described by the respondents. Although many of these might appear quite unremarkable, such as methods of enabling older people to make choices at meal times, and systems of management through which they are able to wear their own clothing, it has been suggested that they do, in fact, make an important contribution to the quality of life of the older person in hospital.

Reference has also been made to the psychological literature on control. Research has been discussed that identifies a clear link between the degree of control available to older people, and their psychological well-being. Furthermore, it has been shown that, despite their enthusiastic approval of the principle of individuality, there are a number of circumstances in which staff feel justified in limiting the choices that older people in hospital care can make. Techniques such as 'coming to a compromise', 'massive encouragement' and 'forcing' have been discussed. Finally, individuality has been linked with Heidegger's concept of existence.

# Chapter 11
# Organising care to promote quality of life

The purposes of this chapter are:

- to describe the general features of an approach to organising nursing care for older people, in hospitals, nursing homes and other settings apart from their own homes, that will promote quality of life;
- to contrast this with an alternative approach that will inhibit quality of life.

Existing literature is drawn into the discussion as and when appropriate; and examples of good (and less good) practice are introduced from the interview transcriptions.

Approaches to organising care in the text tend to fall into one of the two patterns shown in Box 11.1, of which one is inimical to quality of life and one tends to promote it.

## The total institution

Goffman (1961) introduced the concept of the 'total institution' to describe the characteristics of certain places of residence and work where a large number of individuals spend a considerable period of time together, leading an enclosed and formally administered round of life. Its characteristics include:

- rigidity of routine;
- block treatment of residents;
- depersonalisation of residents;
- social distance between residents and staff.

Goffman identified a number of characteristics of the classic institution:

**Box 11.1** Two approaches to organising care

● The first can be called the 'institutional' pattern of care, using a term that frequently appears in the text and is well referenced in the literature of sociology and the caring disciplines.

● The second is less easy to represent epigramatically. Although the word 'home' appears as an obvious choice, I have rejected it because it is often applied to settings where institutional rather than domestic norms prevail, and because I doubt whether it is possible for a nursing home to act as full substitute for the home that it so often replaces. I therefore associate the second pattern of care with a rather clumsy phrase from the data, 'being in the real world'.

1   All aspects of life are conducted in the same place and under the same single authority.

2   Each phase of the member's daily life is conducted in the close company of a large number of others, all treated alike and required to do the same things together.

3   All phases of the day's activities are tightly rostered, with one activity leading at a pre-arranged time into the next. Typically, the whole sequence of events is imposed from above by a body of officials who follow a set of explicit, formal rulings.

4   The various enforced activities are brought together into a single rational plan which is supposed to fulfil the official aims of the institution.

Goffman's theory of the total institution has often been cited in research into the organisation of care for dependent people (Townsend 1962, Baker 1978, Clark and Bowling 1989, Wilkin and Hughes 1987, Hughes and Wilkin 1987, Booth 1985, Willcocks *et al.* 1987, Stacey 1981). Miller and Gwynne's (1972) research into the organisation of residential homes for people with physical handicaps offers a clear picture of the institution at work. Miller and Gwynne argued that the primary task of these homes was to act as warehouses for people who are socially dead until their physical death. The warehousing model is principally concerned with the prolongation of life with little concern for its quality. The emphasis is on cure and the application of medical and nursing care to a passive and dependent patient, who accepts the institution's definition of his or her problems, and strategies for care. The model's main feature is the application of staff-determined routines without regard to the individual characteristics of the patient.

The interview transcription makes frequent reference to institutional patterns of care. In this section, institutional roles, institutional patterns of work and institutional forms of relationship are discussed.

## *The institutional role of patient*

Sister M suggests that two possibilities face the person entering an institutional system in which there is limited opportunity to exercise choice:

*Sister M*: Well, there are two things to not giving the patient choice; first you get a rebellious patient, if they've got . . . what it takes. They'll rebel, and do their damnedest to work against you. Or they'll just become institutionalised: 'Can I go to the toilet, nurse – is it time to go to the toilet, nurse', that kind of thing.
*Researcher*: You said institutionalised. What does that mean?
*Sister M*: Whereby the institution is the most important thing, and they have to conform to the institution's . . .
*Research Assistant*: Routine?
*Sister M*: Right. You'll have your dinner at twelve, you'll go to the toilet at half past, you know . . .

This passage suggests that at an early point, the individual will be faced with institutional life's limitations to choice. Implicit here and more explicit in other parts of the text is the suggestion that the institution has particular goals. Their precise nature will vary according to the purpose of the institution. In the care of older people, they may well be the goals of cure as medically defined, or rapid completion of nursing work. Typically, the goals of the institution take precedence over the goals of the individual ('the institution is the most important thing').

Certain mechanisms exist to encourage the individual to conform to the goals and routine of the institution. These include removal of the element of choice in terms of what will be worn, how the day will be structured and the environment arranged, and so forth. The consequences to the individual of institutionalisation through lack of choice are described by Sister Q:

*Sister Q*: I think . . . probably they'll lose a lot of their identity. I don't think it would be too nice, really. I mean, we do that to some extent now. The patients don't have any choice in meals, the clothing is picked out by nursing staff, and you don't really get to know them as people, do you?

When asked why choice was taken away from people during institutionalisation, Sister K answered:

*Sister K*: Because it's easier for us. It's easier for us to take control and responsibility than to let them have it. I think it's easier. It's easier and quicker for us to make decisions than for us to have to sit down and talk to somebody and allow them to make their own decisions.

Sister L agreed that the physical work of nursing was made a lot easier if patients were denied choice. However, from the point of view of the institution, the removal of choice accomplishes a more important function. As we have seen, the removal of the choice of clothing when a person dresses in hospital attire has ontological significance: it signifies and accomplishes a change in role from person to patient, and serves as a continuing reminder to the person and the institution that such a change has taken place. A person can ask questions, raise objections, disagree, ask for a second opinion, choose not to go to bed, choose not to get out of bed, administer her or his own medication or miss a dose, whereas an institutionalised patient is unlikely to do any of these things, and therefore will present minimal obstacles to the institution in pursuit of its goals.

## *The institutional role of nurse*

Throughout the data there is evidence that the processes of institutionalisation apply to staff as well as to patients, and that the
institutional mode of organisation demands a pattern of behaviour
from nurses that constitutes a role. This role, like that of patient, is
also oriented to the achievement of institutional goals. At times,
pressure to achieve these goals can be overt:

*Sister L*: A lot of the reasons for reducing choice is pressure on
nurses, to get everyone up and dressed and in the dayroom with
no time to talk to anyone. Dr A [the consultant] once gave me a
row for beds not being made, and not everyone being dressed.
He said it wasn't like the days when the old school of nurses was
on duty for a ward round. He is very impressed with everyone
being sat by their beds and washed. It makes me feel very guilty
because I know that everyone will have been got out first thing
and washed and dressed with very little choice, but the consultant likes it.

Aspects of the behaviour of those working within the institutional
role of nurse can be described as routine or ritualistic:

*Sister U*: The longer ones, staff and patients, become very institutionalised, and you can see this if you go into a new area and
staff just do things routinely, and it's very hard to break that routine, because they say, you know, 'We've always done it like this.'

The institutional role of the nurse is reinforced by the uniform.
Respondents suggest that a nurse who wears a uniform will not be
seen as an individual but as a role occupant:

*Sister L*: Unfortunately nurses are stereotyped. A lot of people feel
threatened, you're in uniform, you know what you're doing,
you've been trained. Little do they know! And I think they can
feel very threatened. It's those sorts of barriers that we are starting to break down. They know us by our first names . . . they
know us as people rather than 'the nurse'. I felt it very strongly
when I first came here as a sister. It took me ages even for the
staff to call me [uses first name] . . . I felt it was a big battle I'd
helped to break down, really. After all, you're only a person.

This informant found the uniform an obstacle to her attempts to relate as person to person rather than as nurse to patient. Nevertheless, she was prepared to admit that the uniform could act as emotional armour in the stressful world of nursing.

*Researcher*: Do you think it's important to some nurses, this hiding behind a barrier?

*Sister L*: Yes, probably. I know when I first qualified at sister level, not so much here, but when I was on the acute area, coronary care, reception unit, we had an awful lot of stand-bys, crashes, deaths. At that stage, I found it so much easier that I was in uniform, that I knew what I was saying, explaining; while I felt that if I was out of uniform, I would have cracked up with them. Yes, it was like a pillar. Yes, it did give me a bit of support.

A recurring theme in the context of institutional nursing is that of 'busyness'. Busyness refers to the complexity and pace of nursing work. It emerges in many interviews as mitigation for institutional patterns of care:

*Researcher*: And the staffing levels – do you think they are important?

*Sister L*: Yes, I do. I mean, we're running on six and four [with six staff on the morning and four on the afternoon shift], so even the nurse in charge has got to give hands-on care. Not that I'm against that, but I think you're trying to give the hands-on care, be in charge of the ward, co-ordinate the students, co-ordinate the agency staff – how many hats do you have to wear? You know in that morning, everyone is under pressure, and so the psychological care goes out of the window. I just find myself – awful – you go home and think, 'What have I done this morning?' I even cut conversations short because you know you haven't got time to develop something a patient's trying to tell you, because you haven't got the time to investigate or to dig a bit deeper and find out more about them, and it's not usually until the afternoon that you've got the time to go back to them, and by that time they think you're not interested . . . the telly probably plonked on, Radio One is blaring out and nobody is listening to it, they're all sitting there dozing. I just think it's awful, I really do.

## *Institutional patterns of relationship*

The respondents suggest that the nature of the human relationships experienced by older people has a direct bearing on the quality of their lives:

*Sister T*: Somehow the way we relate to each other is important.
*Researcher*: Yes.
*Sister T*: And most people don't feel happy unless they are in relationships.

Patterns of relationship can be described as either expressive or utilitarian. An expressive pattern of relationship, for the present purpose, is one whose effect is to recognise and confirm the humanity of the other. There is an example in the discussion that followed Sister T's introduction of the concept of social talk:

*Researcher*: Why is social talk important?
*Sister T*: Because – I don't know – because that's what we do. We do talk to people for pleasure and contact, not just to find out information and to give instructions. It's something to do with forming relationships with other people which we need.

Further information is found in the interview with Sister N, who was asked what was important in relationships:

*Sister N*: Things like, as I've said, to be loved, and feeling a part, as it were.
*Researcher*: And how can you do that, something like being loved?
*Sister N*: I think you can. I think it depends on what you mean by love. I don't mean love in marriage particularly, but perhaps being cared for is a more appropriate word, I think. I've got some excellent staff in this day hospital, and I think they do care about the patients.
*Researcher*: Involvement?
*Sister N*: Yes, like I said before, having time to spend with people, and using the time that is there to spend with patients as opposed to sitting in the dayroom drinking coffee.

In contrast, the goal of the utilitarian relationship is to accomplish some task:

*Sister L:* If all your basic needs are met, also your mental needs, it's very important to get to know the person individually, to see what their mental needs are.

The purpose of getting to know people here is 'to see what their mental needs are'. The relationship is constructed with the specific goal of discovering a class of need. While it is clearly legitimate for a nurse–patient relationship to have a task-focused dimension, the text asserts that expressive relationships are also important. However, the expressive dimension is particularly at risk in the institutional pattern of care, where activity is driven by the need to get through the work.

Study of the nature of expressive and utilitarian relationships is informed by Buber's work, summarised in Box 11.2.

---

**Box 11.2 'I–Thou' and 'I–It' relationships**

Buber (1958) writes that there are two primary ways in which one person can relate to another: 'I–Thou', and 'I–It'. In the relationship of I–Thou, each person is 'open' to the other. The other is not regarded as an external object, or as a means to some end, but stands as an end in himself or herself. Macquarrie (1972:110) explains that for Buber, a true relation 'preserves the other in his otherness, and his uniqueness', and that it 'leaves room for him to be himself'. He describes the true relation as a 'dialogical relation', in which each partner is respectfully open to the other without trying to change him or her. Macquarrie describes Buber's insistence on the idea of 'confirmation', which suggests that a person truly becomes himself or herself through the relation to the other. For Buber, there can be no 'I' without a 'Thou'.

---

However, it is equally possible for relationship to take the form 'I–It'. Macquarrie notes that when this occurs we do not relate to another person in wholeness and in openness but turn her or him into a thing, or an instrument. Macquarrie suggests that extreme instances of this are slavery and prostitution, but that it often happens in more subtle ways, wherever there is exploitation or discrimination or prejudice, and persons are treated as less than personal.

Some of the staff , like Sister L (quoted above), claimed that the pressure of work often restricted their interactions with patients to the utilitarian type:

*Sister N*: I've worked on many wards where you do the very basics for people, and there's no time to spend with people, no time to be interested in what they do, what's happening to them at home, how they feel, even to sit down and talk about the weather.

The following quotation suggests that pathology, as well as social structure, has its impact on interpersonal relationships:

*Sister L*: Mrs J is a classic case. She had a severe stroke and her relatives visit every day, and what do they do? They sit at the bottom of the bed and talk among themselves. I'm not saying they don't talk to her, but it's very much a case of 'What do we say to Mother now?' So they just tend to sit there and vegetate.

The final observation to be made about the institutional approach to the organisation of care is that it seems to be context dependent. The institutional roles, patterns of behaviour and relationships described in this and previous chapters seem only able to flourish in a dedicated establishment such as a hospital or nursing home. (See the comments of Sister R, the district nurse cited in Chapter 10, on forcing patients nursed in their own homes.)

The institutional pattern of care is clearly inimical to quality of life, for the reasons shown in Box 11.3.

However, the data also suggest many ways in which staff sought to promote the quality of the lives of older people in their care. Because no word is readily at hand, the phrase 'being in the real world' is introduced from the text to characterise the activities, attitudes and orientation which together are important if care is to be conducive to a life of quality. The nursing home that promotes the older person's 'being in the real world' will not simply act as a warehouse, but will recognise that home is an important locus of

**Box 11.3 Inimical effects of the institutional approach**

Classically, the institutional approach:

- superimposes its own agenda on that of the older person, suppressing self-determination and the expression of choice;
- replaces ontologically significant material artefacts such as clothing and personal possession with functional alternatives;
- reduces human relationship to a utilitarian minimum;
- replaces meaningful activity with idleness.

In each of these ways, the institution undermines the status of the older person as a human being.

personal meaning, and that it represents the 'territorial core' of the social and geographical world.

## Promoting quality of life: being in the real world

*Sister L*: If you're going to be in hospital for a long time and you're not acutely ill, you don't need to be tied to that bed area. I think it's important to see about getting the patient out and seeing the real world.

At the heart of the 'real world' approach to care is the intention to maintain and enhance an individual's capacity to function as a human being. For instance, Sister Q recognised that by the time patients had reached the age of most of hers, they had built up a life and a social structure which could soon be eroded by hospitalisation and would be difficult to rebuild. She felt that it was important to help them maintain contact with their life outside the hospital, as this would help them on discharge. Sister M made a similar point:

*Researcher*: Do you think continuity with normal life is important?
*Sister M*: Yes I do, but it's not always possible.
*Researcher*: Why do you think it's important?

*Sister M*: One thing is it's this attitude thing again, so the patient realises there is something going on outside these four walls, relates to husband, children, grandchildren, all the rest of it. It does keep them in touch with the outside world if they can talk to visitors, see the news, read a newspaper, all these things.

*Researcher*: Remain an individual, not just a patient?

*Sister M*: Yes, Mrs Smith with three tiny grandchildren.

*Researcher*: As opposed to the lady with the stroke in the first bed on the left.

*Sister M*: Yes.

The phrase 'the real world' also reflects the continuing interest that many older patients had in the world beyond the ward doors. For instance, Mr H and Mrs Z simply missed being able to get out and about. Mrs C kept an interest in the prices of food in shops, and professed herself 'Absolutely staggered' at the news that the price of cheese was £1.50 a pound. She added, 'By hell, I can remember the days when you could get the best that was made for one and six-pence a pound.' In a similar way, it was also evident that she enjoyed disparaging the modern music on the radio.

Central to 'real world' care is the belief that one is most likely to enjoy a life of quality without the institutional setting:

*Researcher*: If you could do one thing to improve the quality of the patients' lives on this ward, what would it be?

*Sister K*: Um, I'd knock the four walls down, I wouldn't have the ward, I don't think.

*Researcher*: Right. A bit drastic, I think?

*Sister K*: I don't think I'd have the ward.

*Researcher*: What would you have?

*Sister K*: I'd have everybody I think at home.

Although the recommendation to 'knock the four walls down' may be more rhetorical than realistic, the theme of homeliness persists throughout the text. Several of the caring staff echoed the feeling that a life of quality was most likely in the person's own home. It was because their work enhanced this possibility that the staff from the day hospital felt they made a significant contribution to the care of elderly people:

*Sister N*: It's not really a ward but a day hospital. I think a lot of what we do here to maintain quality of life is to maintain people in the community so that they can choose to go on living at home if that's what they choose to do, instead of being taken to an institution as such. So I think that's a really important part of how we maintain quality of life. And the same goes for, like, carers. We have patients in for a day so carers can have a rest, and perhaps feel fresher and more able to meet their relatives' needs when they go back home, so I think that's really important.

Of course, there are those for whom an independent life in the community is not possible, even with the support of the day hospital. In these cases, the respondents suggest that it is important to make the residence as 'homely' as possible.

Considerable attention was paid to the nature and importance of home in Chapter 9. It was shown that home is an important locus of meaning for many of the older people interviewed, and it was argued that the quality of homeliness is an aspect of the phenomenon of attachment to place, which is itself a characteristic of our being-in-the-world. The discussion explored the following aspects of home:

- physical, social, and autobiographical insideness;
- home as a locus of autonomy;
- personal possessions;
- the continuity of living patterns;
- privacy.

Whether the home is conceptualised as a territory to be defended, a locus of personal control, a zone of self-expression, a reservoir of personal possessions, or playing a part in the self-interpretative processes of human being, there is little doubt that for many people it is a place of great personal significance. If the value of an older person's home depends at all on its particular geographical location, on the social possibilities that it represents and the autobiography that it symbolises, then it is unrealistic to expect that it can easily be recreated in a nursing home. Nevertheless, there are certain principles that ought to be respected if the nursing home is to reflect domestic rather than institutional ideals (Willcocks *et al.* 1987).

The interview transcriptions contain evidence of attempts by the staff to address the various dimensions of homeliness. Particular attention is given to promoting interpersonal relationships and meaningful activity, as shown in the next section. A subsequent section examines aspects of the literature related to this issue.

## *Promoting interpersonal relationships*

The text explores the quality of the relationship between older people in care and their family and friends. Many of the older people interviewed felt that the role of the staff was restricted to the physical aspects of care, and clearly valued visits from family and friends, both for the continuing contact they provided with the real world, and for their own sake:

*Researcher*: When they [your sisters] come and see you, what do you chat about?

*Mrs I*: Oh, all sorts of things, really, that have happened in the past, and things. And where they've been in the morning or afternoon, what they've bought, and one thing and another. Just little everyday things. So like, when you go home from work and you see your mother or your wife or what, well you have your tea and sit down and chat, and little everyday things, don't you? Well, that's what we chat about.

From the perspective of the nursing staff, Sister Q also suggested that the person's quality of life can be enhanced if relatives are involved in care:

*Researcher*: Do you think it improves a patient's quality of life to have relatives involved?

*Sister Q*: Yes, I'm sure it will do.

*Researcher*: Why do you think that is?

*Sister Q*: Because they'll be getting more out of a one-to-one than I can give. With his wife here he's talking about his family, what's been happening, stuff that we don't know, stuff that we can't talk about. We can't go much beyond the weather, what it's like, stuff like that. We might be able to say when she's coming, but we can't add any stuff like about what his son has been doing over the weekend, and other little bits.

The data disclose considerable variation in the amount of care relatives are prepared or able to undertake: some can make a substantial contribution while others are reluctant even to visit. Clearly, there may be many reasons for people's reluctance to involve themselves in care. However, it has been argued that some of those who are able to make a contribution might be inhibited by institutional patterns of care. Sister L was taking deliberate steps to resolve this problem:

*Sister L*: We've got the relatives' action group under way now, and that has been brilliant. And so in many ways because the nurses are under pressure, not only on the ward, but also in trying to get some sort of stimulation, why not get the relatives a bit more involved? Things are already starting to look up. We're trying to devise a better service for relatives on the ward, so it will make them enjoy their visit, and probably encourage them to visit a bit more. So we're trying to improve facilities, like have an area where they can sit and take Mum or Dad out of the area of the bedside or the dayroom.

A number of benefits which may transfer to other care settings were attributed to the meetings of the action group. They are shown in Box 11.4.

---

**Box 11.4 Key benefits of a relatives' action group**

- teaching relatives about the principles underlying care;
- teaching the safe use of equipment such as wheelchairs;
- finding out what the relatives feel about the facilities of the ward, and standards of care;
- relatives understanding how to position people after a stroke;
- identifying various grades of staff to relatives;
- having talks about the roles of different members of the ward team;
- enhancing the relatives' confidence.

Staff also attempted to promote interaction between older people themselves. Sometimes, formal discussion groups were set up:

*Sister L*: The other morning we set up a talk theme about the 1930s, so we set it up and they all sat round, and afterwards, me and Nicky [another member of the nursing team] went in and talked about it. It only took fifteen minutes of nursing time afterwards to discuss how they all felt about it. Even the likes of [names a patient] was talking about a boyfriend she'd got. He was killed in the Second World War. She started to fill up and got really upset. It's a side to [names person again] that you don't see. I mean, because she's demented I sometimes think we treat her like a child.

Some staff also attested to the social aspect of meal times:

*Sister Q*: There are patients who need everything doing for them, feeding. There are others who can maybe use a spoon but perhaps one that might use a knife and fork. So we've got different degrees even among this, so we have the ones who feed themselves sat together, then the ones who maybe need help sat together, and that's to kind of promote something with the ones who are perhaps able to feed themselves, are more presentable, are able to chat with one another. All right, so maybe they can't understand each other, but there is some communication going on there. On another table there are some who are quite active and fight, but there is some interaction there and I feel it's important that that's happening. And as well, when they go sitting in the day-room, if they are not going to communicate you want them looking out so at least they can see you, or they might be sat next to somebody who's going to touch them, or whatever. So we try to do that.

## Promoting meaningful activity

Interviewed patients consistently complained that hospital life was boring. Mrs R was unable to pursue her normal hobby of reading and spent a lot of time looking out of the window instead. Mrs B complained that it was difficult to pass the time, and she too spent time looking out of the window. Similar complaints were made by Mrs I and Mr D. In response, some members of the nursing staff described efforts that they made to stimulate and usefully occupy patients:

*Sister L*: What else do we try to do here? Certainly the activities we do in the afternoon, and try to stimulate any interests they've got. They do get very institutionalised.

*Researcher*: Are they running now, the activities?

*Sister L*: We have got a set programme for Monday to Friday, and then at the weekends, because you don't have the pressure from the rest of the team, the activities are fitted more into what the patients want to do, and not into pigeon holes of what staff we've got and what time we've got, so it's a bit more individual on the weekends.

The next extract from the text identifies several important aspects of the organisation of activity and is therefore reproduced at length:

*Sister N*: I suppose stimulation is quite an important part of what we do to maintain people's quality of life, you know . . . so instead of just sitting around and not really doing anything, we do try and stimulate people into making good use of their faculties that they've still got, to whatever level we can gear it towards. You know, people that are quite confused, it's still important for them to feel that they're achieving something, that they can still answer simple quiz questions.

*Researcher*: I saw your quiz cards in the office.

*Sister N*: Yes, and to work to a higher level for people who aren't confused, just depressed you know, much more difficult things, but still helping them to feel they've achieved something, they've gone through a quiz and been able to answer some questions, they've made some item of craft or whatever, just an end product to say, 'This is what I've done.'

*Researcher*: Yes, at the end of the day, to say, 'I've done this'.

*Sister N*: Yes.

*Researcher*: So what specifically do you do here then?

*Sister N*: Quite a lot of things, really, quite a wide range, because we do gear it to different levels of how people are – like people who are organically ill and people who are functionally ill. There's a very specific difference there, because people come [to the day hospital] on different days depending on which category they're coming into. So on the days it's more organically ill people then it's things like art work, very simple craft work, some reality orientation; but if someone said that to me I'd ask them what they meant, it covers such a wide spectrum of things . . . Just general stimulation about things that have gone by, about the war, how they used to live; but also bringing it back into how they live today in comparison to how they lived in years gone by. And just simple word games like finishing proverbs, and things like that we do for the organically ill.

For the functionally ill we can do much more difficult craft work, some quite intricate sewing, and knitting things; things like collecting rose petals and making scented baskets, things that look really nice, and much more difficult quizzes. We've recently done a really good group on reminiscing about the war, and what people were doing when war was declared, you know; getting down to much more specific things rather than a general discussion.

Several observations can be made about this extract:

1  The staff felt activities were important both as a means of maintaining the abilities of elderly people, and as a way of giving a sense of satisfaction through accomplishment.
2  Efforts were made to tailor the activities to the needs and abilities of the client group, where possible by developing an interest that was already present.
3  There was a wide range of activities from those such as sewing, which demanded practical skills, to those like quizzes and reminiscence, where the emphasis was more on intellectual and social skills.

Activities were not always as formally organised as those described above, but sometimes arose from the everyday interaction of staff and patients. Sister O described a nursing auxiliary who used to sing at the top of her voice and encourage people to sing back to her. Sister O was of the opinion that spontaneous, everyday activities of this type should be included alongside a more carefully planned programme.

# The effects of moving into a nursing home

The consequences for an older person of moving to new accommodation are not easily predicted. A number of studies have focused on mortality rates following relocation. In their literature review, Gutman and Herbert (1976) found evidence that elderly people die at excessively high rates during the first year, and particularly during the first three months following relocation. This applied whether relocation involved movement from the community into a mental hospital, from the community into a residential home for elderly people, from one institution to another, or from one ward to another within the same institution. On the other hand, Coffman (1981) felt two decades of research had only produced equivocal evidence as to whether relocation was likely to affect the survival of older people, and under what conditions. His meta-analysis of twenty-six relocated groups found no general relocation effect, and no systematic effect of age, sex, mental and physical status, choice, preparation, environmental change, or mass versus individual transfer on post-move mortality. He agrees with other researchers that relocation is a significant event in the life of an older person, and conceptualises it in terms of Selye's theory that the level of stress which makes one person sick can be an invigorating experience for another. Coffman observes that the lives of some institutionalised persons are so unstressed that relocation pure and simple would be revitalising, while for others, the stress could prove fatal. Carp (1966) also comments that the outcome of relocation may be anything from total disorganisation and destruction of adaptive capacity to an increased sense of mastery and an improvement in adaptive resources.

The idea that the impact of the stress of relocation will be mediated by its meaning is supported by the interviews. There is evidence that for some older people, the move to a nursing home represents an increased sense of personal safety and confidence, while for others, it represents a disastrous loss of independence. In the management of a nursing home, it would therefore seem logical to tailor the admission procedure to the individual needs of the older person. In the next section, some of the issues of relocation to nursing homes will be discussed with a view to developing standards of practice. The discussion will involve:

- the period preceding the transfer;
- aspects of the move itself;
- the continuity of living patterns;
- the importance of personal possessions;
- privacy.

## The period of preparation for the move

Rutman and Freedman (1988) found that the meaning of home to people in the midst of relocation had never been examined, and therefore took this as their research question. The study was conducted in Toronto, and the sample constituted sixty-three older people who had applied for rent subsidised apartments. The Philadelphia Geriatric Center (PGC) Multilevel Assessment Instrument was used to assess a range of psychosocial and other variables, and open-ended questionnaires were used to explore the meaning of the present home and attitudes to relocation. Each instrument was administered at the time of application for a new apartment and again twelve months later. On the second occasion, approximately one half of the applicants had been relocated.

The finding of particular interest here relates to perceptions of choice and control. Respondents still on the waiting list after one year showed no decline in the variables measured by the PGC Multilevel Instrument, while those who had already completed the move increased their scores on measures of morale, overall psychological adjustment, overall social interaction, mobility, housing, neighbourhood and overall environmental satisfaction. The researchers comment that whereas the traditional literature on the impact of relocation has tended to highlight health and psychological decrements as a function of moving, their own data suggest that the process of moving need not result in declining well-being and performance. They partially attribute their own findings to the fact that 82 per cent of the respondents perceived that they had a degree of control over the relocation process. However, the recency of the move for the relocated group is unreported, and it is possible that their optimistic responses constitute a cognitive restructuring of their situation. Another difficulty with this study is that the respondents involved were relocating to non-institutional accommodation. Nevertheless, the work of Rutman and Freedman offers a degree of empirical support to the ethically based belief that older people should both have and believe themselves to have control over the process of relocation to nursing home accommodation, and this should be reflected in nursing home policy and practice.

## The process of moving to a nursing home

Porteous (1976) paints a grim picture of the process of admission to a nursing home. He suggests that the transfer of a person from their own home to 'euphemistic home' is usually highly traumatic. This trauma is induced not only through the sense of loss of home but also because of the quality of life in institutions. In contrast with the homes their occupants have left, he suggests that euphemistic homes lack warmth and privacy.

It is difficult to know how far this describes reality, because there is little British research on the process of admission into nursing homes. Standards for care must therefore be elaborated from theoretical principles and supported by generalisation from tangentially relevant studies. The contribution of Shulz and Brenner (1977) to the literature of relocation is theoretical rather than empirical. They examined the literature relating to moves from institution to institution, and home to home, and then proposed that an individual's response to the stress of relocation is largely determined by the perceived predictability and controllability of the events surrounding the move, and differences in controllability between pre- and post-relocation environments.

Gutmann and Herbert (1976) examined the impact of relocation on eighty-one male extended-care patients who were moved from an old hospital building due for demolition to a new site. They found that, with the careful preparation of patients, relatives and staff, the mortality rate of their sample was significantly lower than might have been expected.

It is therefore suggested that older people who are preparing for admission to nursing home accommodation should:

- be given information about the events surrounding the move;
- have the opportunity to influence these events through the exercise of choice.

## Continuity of living patterns

In Gutmann and Herbert's (1976) study, care was taken to limit the disruption of the pattern of everyday living following relocation. This finding can logically be applied to the nursing home setting in so far as patterns of living are a function of choice, because it has been shown that home is a locus of autonomy. One would therefore expect a nursing home to possess mechanisms through which the continuity of living patterns could be assured.

## The importance of personal possessions

It has been argued that the objects which the home contains and by which it is in some degree constituted play an important role in the interpretative process of human being (see Chapter 9). It follows that the loss of personal possessions can be one of the most significant aspects of moving into institutional care, and several writers make this point. Carp (1966), for instance, comments that the surrender of furniture and other possessions is very important not only because the objects are missed as items in themselves and as reminders of the family events associated with them, but also because their absence and the substitution of cheaper and less distinguished furnishings is a continual reminder of loss of status.

Frankl (1955) has commented that when all of a person's possessions are taken away, the person has nothing with which to form an external link with her or his former life, and Goffman (1961) has pointed out that in total institutions, the loss of personal possessions prevents the individual from presenting her or his usual image of herself or himself to others.

Kalymun (1983) found that although older people were prepared to reduce the amount of their belongings when relocating, bringing part of their former lives with them in the form of personal objects helped them to feel emotionally whole. Schmitt *et al.* (1977) found more significant and optimal functioning in elderly people who took transitional objects from their old homes into nursing homes, and Altman (1975) noted that people in hospital are comforted by having personal objects about them which serve as reminders of home. This evidence suggests that encouraging individuals to retain personal possessions when moving into an institutional setting will make a positive outcome more likely. As Furby (1978) comments, it is as if possessions permit a healthy degree of personal control or competence in a relatively uncontrollable environment and thereby foster positive attitudes and adaptive behaviour.

## *The importance of privacy*

Control of access to the home environment is made possible through the definition and defence of territorial boundaries. Respect for these boundaries reflects the function of the home as a zone of personal autonomy. There is evidence that access to private dwelling space is the typical expectation of older people in Britain today. Willcocks *et al.* (1987) observe that the majority of the very old (80-plus) live in their own houses in the community, and one half of these live alone. Only 2 per cent of those aged 80–84 and 5 per cent of those aged over 85 have non-relatives in their households. The policies and practices of the nursing home should therefore demonstrate respect for privacy.

## Summary

This chapter has described two types of approach to the management of care in nursing homes: the institutional, which undermines quality of life, and an alternative approach that will tend to promote it. In the next chapter, some of the implications of the eudaemonistic approach to quality of life are discussed.

# Chapter 12

# Conclusion: quality of life and its contribution to nursing practice

The purpose of this closing chapter is:

- to summarise briefly the arguments and the evidence that have been presented;
- to make concluding statements about the significance of the concept of quality of life for our understanding of contemporary nursing practice and patient well-being.

Asked to describe the goals of nursing care in general terms, many nurses would volunteer, or at least agree with the suggestion, that they work to promote the quality of life of their patients and clients. They would probably use the term 'quality of life' in the same rather general sense in which it is commonly used in everyday life by professionals and lay people alike. This common meaning is difficult to define crisply and clearly, but it has a rather positive feel to it and carries overtones of 'helping people to achieve their potential', 'doing what is best' for them, 'promoting their well-being'. This would lead one to suppose that nurses possess practical and research-based knowledge about circumstances and strategies in and through which patients' quality of life can be enhanced, and in fact, the nursing literature contains a good deal of information of this kind. However, very little of this literature is specifically concerned with the meaning of quality of life. Furthermore, it tends not to employ the concept explicitly either as a source of ideas or as a 'gold standard' against which to compare extant practice.

This book is based on the assumption that a clearly defined and explicitly stated concept of quality of life might help us to evaluate aspects of current nursing practice, and might also enable us to generate new ideas for organising patient care. We have attempted to provide the outline for such a theory.

The book began with a literature review. Although 'quality of life' is probably one of the currently most widely used phrases in the English language, it is impossible to ascribe a single, definitive meaning to it. In fact, its meaning changes from one body of literature to another. This does not automatically constitute a problem, because we know that the meanings of concepts tend to evolve as they are put to various uses at different times and in different places (Rodgers and Knafl 1993); and despite an apparent lack of definition, there is clearly a pattern in the way the concept of quality of life is used in the health-related literature.

We began to see the first outlines of this pattern in our review of the social indicators literature. The early literature is important because it represents the first attempt to use the concept of quality of life in a systematic way, and so sets the scene for later work in other fields. Three important points can be made about this literature, as shown in Box 12.1.

---

**Box 12.1 Key points of the social indicators literature**

- It regards the quality of life as something that can be measured.
- It proposes to measure the quality of life in order to evaluate economic and political policy.
- It is split between the advocates of subjective and objective approaches to measurement.

---

These three elements of measurement, evaluation and the subjective–objective debate are also present in the literature relating quality of life to health in various ways. We have considered two aspects of this literature in some detail:

- QALYs;
- research using quality of life as an outcome in the evaluation of medical treatments.

The element of measurement assumes that the quality of life is present to a greater or lesser extent and that its degree of presence or absence can adequately and reliably be represented by numbers. In all parts of the literature reviewed, there is evidence that considerable effort and ingenuity are expended in developing quality of life measurement scales. Some have very respectable psychometric credentials, while others are rather more crude in design; but whatever their degree of sophistication, it is extremely rare for the assumption that the quality of life can be measured to be challenged or even seriously questioned.

The second common element in the literature is that measurements of the quality of life are frequently given an evaluative role. In social indicators research, the subject of evaluation is the outcome of economic and political policies. In the medical literature, interventions such as surgical operations and drug regimes are evaluated in terms of their effect on patients' quality of life. The QALY is an exception to this rule, for in QALY research, numerical representations of quality of life are combined with other data to assist in making decisions about the allocation of scarce resources. In most cases, measures of quality of life are used inclusively, with the assumed goal of increasing the quality of people's lives, but the QALY uses the concept exclusively, with the purpose of identifying people whose condition is such that further improvements in the quality of life are unlikely, in order to exclude them from access to the health care resource.

The final common element identified in our review is the debate between those who regard the quality of life as an objective phenomenon, and those who consider it to be subjective in nature. Discussing the concept of quality of life with other nurses, I have often found that they advocate a subjective approach. They think that the components of a life of quality vary from person to person and that it would be paternalistic for a nurse to try to guess the things that would please or satisfy another person. It is interesting to note that my own research found a very low level of disagreement between respondents about the elements of a life of quality.

This book has argued that the frequency with which the elements of measurement, evaluation and the subjective–objective debate occur throughout the literature is not an accident, but a result of the common philosophical assumptions each of these approaches to quality of life is based on. Specifically, they share an orientation to the social world that is grounded in positivism. Positivist approaches to the quality of life are basically scientific in nature, and underpinned by a coherent set of beliefs that share the unquestioning approval of many health care practitioners and researchers. Despite this, our review has shown that a significant proportion of the published research does not conform to the highest scientific standards. For instance, medical outcomes researchers often employ quality of life scales of dubious validity and questionable reliability, and their experimental designs are sometimes poorly thought out. Our review has also shown that professionals and some philosophers with an interest in health have expressed reservations about the QALY and its use in the allocation of health service resources.

Although the scientific, positivist approach to the quality of life appears ubiquitous in the contemporary literature, other approaches can be found that are underpinned by alternative philosophical perspectives. One such is the eudaemonistic approach, which takes its name from the ancient Greek word '*eudaemonia*'. As we have seen, this has traditionally been translated as 'happiness', but in the contemporary literature tends to be rendered as 'human flourishing'.

At the heart of the eudaemonistic approach to the quality of life is a view of the nature of human beings. Historically, the positivistic view of the human being has been extremely influential. However, alternative perspectives can be found, and for many decades, antipositivist philosophers and social scientists have debated with positivist scholars on the nature of human beings, and the research methods by which we can understand their social lives. Philosophical hermeneutics is an important school in the antipositivist tradition, and Heidegger one of its most important students in the twentieth century. His account of the nature of human beings emphasises the role that meaning plays in people's lives. He argued that the daily human experience of the world does not correspond with the 'objective' preoccupations of the scientist, but that we usually relate to things in terms of their significance and relevance to our current projects and concerns. Qualitative researchers have found the concept formed by Gadamer (Heidegger's pupil) of 'understanding as the fusion of horizons' of particular value.

Whereas the positivist approach tends to regard the quality of life as an empirical issue that involves the collection of statistical data, the eudaemonistic tends more to regard it as a philosophical problem. Quality of life is related to one's status as a human being. It may seem, of course, that to define the quality of life in terms of human being is simply to replace one difficult concept with another; but as we have seen, a number of philosophical schools have made explicit statements about the nature of human beings, and their work can help us to understand the meaning of quality of life. The eudaemonistic approach is concerned with the nature of the human being, and seeks to identify the circumstances in which human beings are most likely to flourish. I have argued that this approach to the quality of life is more relevant to the everyday work of many nurses than is the scientific approach with its emphasis on measurement and evaluation, as a good deal of nursing work is concerned with creating the circumstances in which human beings can flourish and strive to reach their potential. One area in which this role is clearly seen is in the nursing care of older people in hospital, as rehabilitation from stroke, for instance, involves promoting the older person's independence. Similarly, nursing care in the day hospital setting which enables the older person to remain in his or her home also contributes to quality of life.

In this book, philosophical hermeneutics has provided a methodological tool for the analysis of qualitative interviews, and the hermeneutical perspective on the nature of human beings has provided a framework on which a wide range of relevant literature, and original research by the author, has been organised into a coherent whole. It has provided an account of quality of life that values and explains the significance of ordinary aspects of the human experience such as places, personal possessions and clothing. This account has been related to nurses' descriptions of the measures they take to safeguard and promote the quality of life of older patients in hospital, and it has also been linked to a discussion of the likely impact of different approaches to the organisation of care. We have seen that nurses' actions can either promote or undermine older people's quality of life. Some actions clearly serve to promote their status as human beings. Frequently, these actions involve commonplace activities such as providing a choice, or creating systems of care in which this provision is possible. Examples include enabling the older patient in hospital to continue wearing his or her own clothing, because clothing is an important marker of personal identity, and the provision of a range of appropriate recreational activities throughout the day.

The eudaemonistic approach demonstrates that simple nursing actions of this kind make an important contribution to the quality of life. Equally, however, we have seen that familiar actions may also serve to undermine the status of the person as a human being, challenge her or his individuality, and thereby threaten the quality of her or his life.

In this book, an attempt has been made to classify forms of organisation of the nursing care of older people into ideal types, which vary according to how far they promote the older people's status as human beings. Generations of researchers (Baker 1978, Miller and Gwynne 1972) have demonstrated that the institutional approach to the management of care is invidious. The personal choices that mark individuality give way to batch treatment, and significant personal possessions such as clothing are replaced by forms of dress chosen for their practical utility. Downgrading of the person's individuality in this way is often followed by disrespectful treatment of the person, and can lead to abuse of the kind whose logical extremity is described by Robb (1967).

In the alternative approach to organising care, steps are taken to safeguard patient choice and individuality and promote and support the older person in his or her humanity. Ideally, this involves enabling the older person to be surrounded and supported by significant objects and providing opportunities for choice in daily life. It is unlikely, of course, that even the best-motivated and most able of nurses will ever be able to recreate a place that fully reflects the older person's own home in terms of its significance and meaning, but the research described above has offered ample evidence that many nursing staff are well aware of the importance of home to the older person, and strive to promote individuality and offer choice in a range of care settings.

# References

Abrams, M. (1976) *A Review of Subjective Social Indicators Work: 1971–1975*, London: Social Science Research Council.

Agnew, J. and Duncan, S. (1989) *The Power of Place: Bringing Together Geographical and Sociological Imaginations*, Boston: Unwin Hyman.

Aiken, W. (1982) 'Quality of life', *Philosophy* Spring, 26–36.

Altman, I. (1975) *The Environment and Social Behaviour*, Monterey, CA: Brooks/Cole.

Andrews, F. (1974) 'Social indicators of perceived life quality', *Social Indicators Research* 1, 279–99.

Andrews, F. and Withey, S. (1976) *Social Indicators of Well-being: American Perceptions of Life Quality*, New York: Plenum Press.

Arling, G., Harkins, E. and Capitman, J. (1986) 'Institutionalisation and personal control', *Research on Aging* 8 (1): 38–56.

Averill, J. (1973) 'Personal control over aversive stimuli and its relationship to stress', *Journal of Personality and Social Psychology* 44 (6): 1284–96.

Baker, D. (1978) 'Attitudes of nurses to care of the elderly', unpublished PhD thesis, University of Manchester.

Bakker, C. and van der Linden, S. (1995) 'Health related utility measurement: an introduction', *Journal of Rheumatology* 22 (6): 1197–9.

Bandura, A. (1977) 'Self-efficacy: toward a unifying theory of behaviour change', *Psychological Review* 84: 191–215.

Banziger, G. and Roush, S. (1983) 'Nursing homes for the birds: a control relevant intervention with bird-feeders', *Gerontologist* 32 (5): 527–31.

Barrett, B. and Sloan, T. (1988) 'Critical notes on Packer's Hermeneutic Inquiry', *American Psychologist* Feb.: 131–2.

Bauman, Z. (1978) *Hermeneutics and Social Science*, London: Hutchinson.

de Beauvoir, S. (1973) *The Coming of Age*, New York: Warner.

Benner, P. (1985) 'Quality of life: explanation, prediction and understanding in nursing science', *Advances in Nursing Science* 1: 1–14.

Benner, P. and Wrubel, J. (1989) *The Primacy of Caring: Stress and Coping in Health and Illness*, Menlo Park: Addison-Wesley.

Benner, P., Tanner, C. and Chesla, C. (1992) 'From beginner to expert: gaining a differentiated world in critical care nursing', *Advances in Nursing Science* 14 (3): 13–28.

Bernstein, R. (1983) *Beyond Objectivism and Relativism*, Oxford: Blackwell.

Booth, T. (1985) 'Institutional regimes and resident outcomes for the elderly', in C. Philipson, C. Bernard and P. Strong (eds), *Dependency and Interdependency in Old Age: Theoretical Perspectives and Policy Alternatives*, London: Croom Helm.

Bourdieu, P. (1977) *Outline of a Theory of Practice*, Cambridge: Cambridge University Press.

Bowling, A. (1991) *Measuring Health: a Review of Quality of Life Measurement Scales*, Milton Keynes: Open University Press.

Bradburn, N. and Noll, C. (1969) *The Structure of Psychological Well-Being*, Chicago: Aldine.

Bryckzynski, K. (1989) 'An interpretative study describing the clinical judgement of nurse practitioners'. *Scholarly Inquiry for Nursing Practice* 3 (2): 75–104.

Buber, M. (1958) *I and Thou*, trans R.G. Smith, 2nd edn, New York: Charles Scribners Sons.

Buhl, K., Lehnert, T., Schlag, K. and Herforth, C. (1995) 'Reconstruction after gastrectomy and quality of life', *World Journal of Surgery* 19 (4): 558–64.

Bunge, M. (1975) 'What is a quality of life indicator?', *Social Indicators Research* 2: 65–79.

Bunge, M. (1993) 'Realism and antirealism in social science', *Theory and Decision* 35 (3): 207–35.

Burrell, G. and Morgan, G. (1979) *Sociological Paradigms and Organisational Analysis*, Aldershot: Gower, Heinemann.

Callebaut, W. (1978) 'Social indicators research and the theory of collective action', *Philosophica* 21: 159–97.

Callebaut, W. (1980) 'Philosophical aspects of social indicators and quality of life research', *Philosophica* 26 (2): 161–77.

Campbell, A., Converse, P. and Rogers, W. (1976) *The Quality of American Life*, New York: Russell Sage Foundation.

Campbell, D. and Stanley, J. (1966) *Experimental and Quasi-Experimental Designs for Research*, Chicago: Rand McNally.

Cantril, H. (1965) *Pattern of Human Concerns*, New Brunswick, NJ: Rutgers University Press.

Carley, M. (1981) *Social Measurement and Social Indicators: Issues of Policy and Theory*, London: George Allen and Unwin.

Carp, G. (1966) *A Future for the Aged: Victoria Plaza and its Residents*, Austin, TX: University of Texas Press.

Carr-Hill, R. (1991) 'Allocating resources to health care: is the QALY a technical solution to a political problem?', *International Journal of Health Services* 21 (2): 351–63.

Chowdhary, U. (1990) 'Notion of control and self-esteem in institutionalised men', *Perceptual and Motor Skills* 70: 731–8.

Cicirelli, V. (1987) 'Locus of control and patient role adjustment of the elderly in acute care hospitals', *Psychology and Aging* 2 (2): 138–43.

Clark, P. and Bowling, A. (1989) 'Observational study of quality of life in NHS nursing homes and a long-stay ward for the elderly', *Aging and Society* 9(1): 73–7.

Coffman, T. (1981) 'Relocation and survival of institutionalised aged: a re-examination of the evidence', *Gerontologist* 21 (5): 483–500.

Cohen, L. and Manion, L. (1989) *Research Methods in Education* 3rd edn, London: Routledge.

Cooper, D. (1992) *Existentialism*, Oxford: Blackwell.

Cordwell, J. and Schwarz, R. (1979) (eds) *The Fabrics of Culture: The Anthropology of Clothing and Adornment*, The Hague: Mouton.

Cormack, D. (1990) Editorial: 'The therapeutic influence of the environment: a *nursing* home or a nursing *home*', *Journal of Gerontological Nursing* 16 (3): 3–4.

Crisp, R. (1989) 'Deciding who will die: QALYs and political theory', *Politics* 9 (1): 31–5.

Culyer, A. (1984) 'The quest for efficiency in the public sector: economists versus Dr Pangloss', in *Public Finance and the Quest for Efficiency: Proceedings of the 38th Congress of the International Institute of Public Finance*, Detroit: Wayne State University Press.

Currie, I., Wilson, Y., Baird, R., and Lamont, P. (1995) 'Treatment of intermittent claudication: the impact on quality of life', *European Journal of Vascular and Endovascular Surgery* 10 (3): 356–61.

Dagnan, D., Look, R., Ruddick, L. and Jones, J. (1995) 'Changes in the quality of life of people with learning disabilities who have moved from hospital to community based homes', *International Journal of Rehabilitation Research* 18 (2): 115–22

Dahlof, M. (1991) 'Well-being (quality of life) in connection with hypertension treatment', *Clinical Cardiology* 14 (Feb.): 97–103.

Davis, L. and Lennon, L. (1988) 'Social cognition and the study of clothing and human behaviour', *Social Behaviour and Personality* 16 (2): 175–86.

Den Uyl, D. and Machan, T. (1983) 'Recent work on the concept of happiness', *American Philosophical Quarterly* 20 (2): 115–32.

DeSanto, L., Olsen, D., Perry, W., Rohe, D. and Keith, R. (1995) 'Quality of life after surgical treatment of cancer of the larynx', *Annals of Otology, Rhinology and Laryngology* 104 (10, pt 1): 763–9.

Descartes, R. (1986) *Meditations on First Philosophy*, trans J. Cottingham, Cambridge: Cambridge University Press.

Dey, I. (1993) *Qualitative Data Analysis: A User Friendly Guide for Social Scientists*, London: Routledge.

Diekelmann, N. (1992) 'Learning as testing: a Heideggerian hermeneutic analysis of the lived experience of students and teachers in nursing', *Advances in Nursing Science* 14 (3): 72–83.

Diener, E. (1984) 'Subjective well being', *Psychological Bulletin* 95: 542–75.

Diener, E. (1993) 'Assessing subjective well-being: progress and opportunities', *Social Indicators Research* 31: 103–57.

Donaldson, C., Atkinson, A., Bond, C. *et al.* (1988) 'Should QUALYs be programme specific?', *Journal of Health Economics* 7: 239–57.

Dovey, K. (1978) 'Home: an ordering principle in space', *Landscape* 22: 27–30.

Draper, P. (1994) 'Promoting the quality of life of elderly people in nursing home care: a hermeneutical approach', unpublished PhD thesis, University of Hull.

Dreyfus, H. (1991) *Being-in-the-World: A Commentary on Heidegger's Being and Time, Division One*, Cambridge, MA: MIT Press.

Eagleton, T. (1983) *Literary Theory*, Minneapolis: University of Minneapolis Press.

Elkington, J. (1966) 'Medicine and the quality of life', *Annals of Internal Medicine* 64 (3): 711–14.

Eriksen, M. and Sirgy, M. (1992) 'Employed females' clothing preference, self-image congruence, and career anchorage', *Journal of Applied Social Psychology* 22 (5): 408–22.

Fawcett, J. (1989) *Analysis and Evaluation of Conceptual Models of Nursing* 2nd edn, Philadelphia, PA: F.A. Davis.

Fayers, P. and Jones, D. (1983) 'Measuring and analysing quality of life in cancer clinical trials: a review', *Journal of Statistics in Medicine* 2: 429–46.

Festinger, L. (1957) *Theorie der kognitiven dissonanz (Theory of Cognitive Dissonance)*, Stuttgart: Huber.

Folkman, S. (1984) 'Personal control and stress and coping processes: a theoretical analysis', *Journal of Personality and Social Psychology* 46 (4): 839–52.

Frankl, V. (1955) *The Doctor and the Soul*, New York: Bantam Books.

Freitas, C., Oliveiras, B., Marques, E. and Leite, E. (1995) 'Effect of photorefractive keratectomy on visual functioning and quality of life', *Journal of Refractive Surgery* 11 (3), Suppl. s, 327–34

Furby, L. (1978) 'Possessions: towards a theory of their meaning and function throughout the life-cycle', in P. Baltes (ed.) *Life-span Development and Behaviour*, vol. D, New York: Academic Press.

Gadamer, H. (1975) *Truth and Method*, London: Sheed and Ward.

Geelhoed, E., Harris, A. and Prince, R. (1994) 'Cost-effectiveness analysis of hormone replacement therapy and lifestyle intervention for hip fractures', *Australian Journal of Public Health* 18 (2): 153–60.

Gehrmann, F. (1978) '"Valid" empirical measurement of quality of life?', *Social Indicators Research* 1: 73–110.

Giddens, A. (1976) *New Rules of Sociological Method*, London: Hutchinson.

Gifford, R. (1987) *Environmental Psychology: Principles and Practice*, Boston: Allyn and Bacon.

Giorgi, A. (1975) 'An application of phenomenological method in psychology', in A. Giorgi, C. Fischer and E. Murray (eds) *Duquesne Studies in Phenomenological Psychology*, vol. II, Pittsburgh: Duquesne University Press.

Glaser, B. and Strauss, A. (1967) *The Discovery of Grounded Theory: Strategies for Qualitative Research*, Chicago: Aldine Press.

Goffman, E. (1961) *Asylums: On the Social Situations of Mental Patients and Other Inmates*, Garden City, NY: Anchor Books.

Gould, D. (1975) 'Some lives cost too dear', *New Statesman* 90 (2331): 633–5.

Graham, G. (1990) *Living the Good Life: An Introduction to Moral Philosophy*, New York: Paragon House.

Gross, B. (1966) 'The state of the nation: social systems accounting', in R. Bauer (ed.) *Social Indicators*, Cambridge, MA: MIT Press.

Gudex, C. (1986) 'QALYs and their use in the health service', *Discussion Paper 20*, York: Centre for Health Economics, University of York.

Gudex, C. and Kind, P. (1989) 'The QALY tool kit', *Discussion Paper 38*, York: Centre for Health Economics, University of York.

Guignon, C. (1992) 'History and commitment in the early Heidegger', in H. Dreyfus and H. Hall (eds) *Heidegger: A Critical Reader*, Oxford: Blackwell.

Gutman, G. and Herbert, C. (1976) 'Mortality rates among extended-care patients', *Journal of Gerontology* 31: 352–7.

Haddorn, D. (1991) 'The Oregon priority-setting exercise', *Hastings Center Report* May–June: 11–23.

Harman, H. and Harman, S. (1989) *No Place Like Home: A Report on the First 96 Cases of the Registered Homes Tribunal*, London: NALGO.

Harris, J. (1987) 'QALYfying the value of life', *Journal of Medical Ethics* 13: 117–23.

Harris, J. (1988) 'More and better justice', in J. Bell and S. Mendes (eds) *Philosophy and Medical Welfare*, Royal Institute of Philosophy Lecture Series 23, Supplement to *Philosophy* (1988), Cambridge: Cambridge University Press.

Hayry, M. (1991) 'Measuring the quality of life: why, how and what?' *Theoretical Medicine* 12 (2): 97–116.

Heidegger, M. (1962) *Being and Time*, trans J. Macquarrie and E. Robinson, New York: Harper and Row.

Hekman, S. (1984) 'Action as a text: Gadamer's hermeneutics and the social scientific analysis of action', *Journal for the Theory of Social Behaviour* 14 (3 October): 333–54.

Hekman, S. (1986) *Hermeneutics and the Sociology of Knowledge*, Notre Dame, IN: University of Notre Dame Press.

Hickson, J., Housley, W. and Boyle, C. (1988) 'The relationship of locus of control, age, and sex to life satisfaction and death anxiety in older persons', *International Journal of Aging and Human Development* 26 (3): 191–200.

Hollenberg, N., Testa, M. and Williams, G. (1991) 'Quality of life as a therapeutic end-point: analysis of therapeutic trials in hypertension', *Journal of Drug Safety* 6 (2): 83–93.

Honey, K. (1987) 'The interview as text: hermeneutics considered as a model for analysing the clinically informed research interview', *Human Development* 30, 69–82.

Hughes, B. and Wilkin, D. (1987) 'Physical care and quality of life in residential homes', *Aging and Society* 7, 399–425.

Huxley, P. (1986) *Quality Measurement in Mental Health Services: A*

*Discussion Paper on Quality of Life Measurement*, London: Good Practices in Mental Health.

Jachuk S. and Brierly H. (1982) 'The effect of hypotensive drugs on the quality of life', *Journal of the Royal College of General Practitioners* 32, 103–5.

Johnson, J. (1975) 'Stress reduction through sensory information', in G. Saranson and C. Spielberger (eds) *Stress and Anxiety*, vol. 2, New York: Wiley.

Jones, S. (1985) 'Analysis of depth interviews', in R. Walker (ed.) *Applied Qualitative Research*, London: Gower.

Kaiser, S. (1990) *The Social Psychology of Clothing*, 2nd edn, New York: Macmillan.

Kalymun, M. (1983) 'Factors influencing elderly women's decisions concerning living-room items during relocation' *EDRA: Environmental Design Research Association* 14, 75–83.

Kamlet, M., Paul, N., Greenhouse, J., Kupfer, D., Frank, E. and Wade, M. (1995) 'Cost utility analysis of maintenance treatment for recurrent depression', *Controlled Clinical Trials* 16 (1): 17–40.

Kennedy, L., Northcott, H. and Kinzel, C. (1978) 'Subjective evaluation of well-being: problems and prospects', *Social Indicators Research* 5: 457–74.

Kerlinger, F. (1973) *Foundations of Behavioral Research*, 2nd edn, New York: Holt, Reinhart and Winston.

Kiebert, G., Stiggelbout, A., Kievit, J., Leer, J., van de Velde, C. and de Haes, H. (1994) 'Choices in oncology: factors that influence patients' treatment preference', *Quality of Life Research* 3 (3): 175–82.

King, I. (1981) *A Theory for Nursing: Systems, Concepts, Process*, New York: Wiley.

Kisiel, T. (1969) 'The happening of tradition: the hermeneutics of Gadamer and Heidegger', *Man and World* 2 (3): 358–85.

Kozma, A. and Stones, M. (1988) 'Social desirability in measures of subjective well-being: age comparisons', *Social Indicators Research* 1: 1–14.

Kuhn, T.S. (1970) *The Structure of Scientific Revolutions*, Chicago: University of Chicago Press.

Kumar, P., Zehr, K., Chang, A., Cameron, D. and Baumgartner, W. (1995) 'Quality of life in octogenarians after open heart surgery', *Chest* 108 (4), 919–26.

Kurz, D. and Nunley, M. (1994) 'Ideology and work at Teotihuacan: a hermeneutic approach', *Man* 28, 761–78.

Kvale, S. (1985) 'The qualitative research interview: a phenomenological and hermeneutic mode of understanding', *Journal of Phenomenological Psychology* 14 (2), 171–96.

Kwon, Y. and Farber, A. (1992) 'Attitudes towards appropriate clothing in perception of occupational attributes', *Perceptual and Motor Skills* 74: 163–8.

Langer, E. (1983) 'Introduction: the psychology of control', in E. Langer, *The Psychology of Control*, Beverley Hills: Sage.

Langer, E. and Rodin, J. (1976) 'The effects of choice and enhanced personal responsibility for the aged: a field experiment in an institutional setting', *Journal of Personality and Social Psychology* 34 (2): 191–8.

Larson, R. (1978) 'Thirty years' research on the subjective well-being of older Americans', *Journal of Gerontology* 31: 109–25.

Lazarsfeld, E. (1961) 'Notes on the history of quantification in sociology: trends, sources and problems', in H. Woolf (ed.) *Quantification: A History of the Meaning of Measurement in the Natural and Social Sciences*, Indianapolis: Bobbs-Merrill.

Lefcourt, H. (1982) *Locus of Control: Current Trends in Theory and Research*, Hillsdale, NJ: Erlbaum.

Lehman, A. (1993) 'The effects of psychiatric symptoms on quality assessments among the chronic mentally ill', *Evaluation and Program Planning* 6, 143–51.

Ley, D. (1977) 'Social geography and the taken-for-granted world', *Transactions of the Institute of British Geography* 2: 498–512.

Lim, A., Brandon, A., Fielder, J., Brickman, A., Boyer, C., Raub, W. and Soloway, M. (1995) 'Quality of life: radical prostatectomy versus radiation therapy for prostate cancer', *Journal of Urology* 154 (4): 1420–5.

Linge, D. (1976) Editor's introduction, in H. Gadamer, *Philosophical Hermeneutics*, Berkeley, CA: University of California Press.

Liu, B. (1975) 'Quality of life: concept, measure and results', *American Journal of Economics and Sociology* 34 (1): 1–13.

Loomes, G. and McKenzie, L. (1989) 'The use of QALYs in health care decision making', *Social Science and Medicine* 28 (4): 299–308.

Lukermann, F. (1961) 'The concept of location in classical geography', *Annals (Association of American Geographers)* 57: 194–210.

Lukes, S. (1973) *Individualism*, Oxford: Blackwell.

McCall, S. (1980) 'What is quality of life?' *Philosophica* 25 (1): 5–14.

McIntyre, P., Hall, J. and Leeder, S. (1994) 'An economic analysis of alternatives for childhood immunization against haemophilus-influenza type-b disease', *Australian Journal of Public Health* 18 (4): 394–400.

Macquarrie, J. (1972) *Existentialism: An Introduction, Guide and Assessment*, London: Penguin.

Malcolm-Gill, W. (1984) 'Subjective well-being: properties of an instrument for measuring this in the chronically ill', *Social Science and Medicine* 18 (8): 683–91.

Mancini, J. (1987) 'Effects of control and income on control orientation and life satisfaction among aged public housing residents', *International Journal of Aging and Human Development* 12 (3): 215–20.

Martin, P., Hammersley, M. and Atkinson, P. (1984) *Ethnography Project Guide DE 801*, Milton Keynes: Open University Press.

Maslow, A.H. (1954) *Motivation and Personality*, New York: Harper.

Mason, R. and Faulkenberry, D. (1978) 'Aspiration, achievement and life-satisfaction', *Social Indicators Research* 5: 133–50.

May, C., Smith, P., Murdock, C. and Davis, M. (1995) 'The impact of the implantable cardioverter on quality of life', *Pacing and Clinical Electrophysiology* 18 (7): 1411–18.

Meleis, A. (1991) *Theoretical Nursing: Development and Progress*, 2nd edn, New York: Lippincott.

Melosh, B. (1982) *The Physician's Hand: Work, Culture and Conflict in American Nursing*, Philadelphia, PA: Temple University Press.

Miles, M. and Huberman, M. (1994) *Qualitative Data Analysis: An Expanded Source Book*, 2nd edn, London: Sage.

Mill, J.S. (1879) Chapters on socialism, in *Collected Works*, vol. V, Toronto and London: University of Toronto Press.

Miller, E. and Gwynne, G. (1972) *A Life Apart: A Pilot Study of Residential Institutions for the Physically Handicapped and the Young Chronic Sick*, London: Tavistock Institute of Human Relations, Lippincott.

Miller, S. (1979) 'Controllability and human stress: method, evidence and theory', *Behaviour Research and Therapy* 17: 287–304.

Miller, S. and Combs, C. (1989) 'Information, coping and control in patients undergoing surgery; and stressful medical procedures', in A. Steptoe and A. Appels (eds) *Stress, Personal Control and Health*, Chichester: Wiley.

Moberg, D. and Brusek, P. (1978) 'Spiritual well-being: a neglected subject in quality of life research', *Social Indicators Research* 5: 303 23.

Moore, D. and Schulz, N. (1987) 'Loneliness among the elderly: the role of perceived responsibility and control', *Journal of Social Behaviour and Control* 2: 215–24.

Mulkay, M., Ashmore, M. and Pinch, T. (1987) 'Measuring quality of life: a sociological invention concerning the application of economics to health care', *Sociology* 21 (4): 541–64.

Myken, P., Caidahl, K., Larsson, P., Larsson, S., Wallentin, I. and Berggren, H. (1995) 'Mechanical versus biological valve prosthesis: a ten-year comparison regarding function and quality of life', *Annals of Thoracic Surgery* 60 (2), Suppl. s: 447–52.

Najman, J. and Levine, S. (1981) 'Evaluating the impact of medical care and technologies on quality of life: a review and critique', *Social Science and Medicine* 15: 107–15.

Nord, E. (1993) 'The relevance of health state after treatment in prioritising between different patients', *Journal of Medical Ethics* 19: 37–42.

Nord, E., Richardson, J., Street, A., Kuhse, H. and Singer, P. (1995) 'Who cares about cost? Does economic analysis impose or reflect social values?' *Health Policy* 134 (2): 79–94

O'Bryant, S. (1982) 'The value of home to older persons: relationship to housing satisfaction', *Research on Aging* 4 (3), 349–63.

Olson, G. and Schober, B. (1993) 'The satisfied poor: development of an intervention oriented theoretical framework to explain satisfaction with a life in poverty', *Social Indicators Research* 28: 173–93.

Orth-Gomer, K., Britton, M. and Rehnquist, N. (1979) 'Quality of care in an outpatient department: the patient's view', *Social Science and Medicine* 13A: 347–57.

Page, C. (1991) 'Philosophical hermeneutics and its meaning for philosophy', *Philosophy Today* Summer: 127–36.

Palmer, R. (1969) *Hermeneutics: Interpretation Theory in Schleiermacher, Dilthey, Heidegger and Gadamer*, Evanston, IL: Northwestern University Press.

Palmer, T. (1987) 'Gadamer's hermeneutics and social theory', *Critical Review* Summer: 91–108.

Palmore, E., Brusse, E., Maddox, G., Nowlin, G. *et al.* (1985) *Normal Aging III*, Durham: Duke University Press.

Paton, C. (1995) *Health Policy and Management: The Health Care Agenda in a British Political Context*, London: Chapman Hall.

Peschar, J. (1977) *The Social Distribution of Life-space*, Groningen: Institute of Sociology, University of Groningen.

Peters, T. (1974) 'The nature and role of presupposition: an inquiry into contemporary hermeneutics', *International Philosophical Quarterly* 14: 209–22.

Phull, P., Ryder, S., Halliday, D., Price, A., Levi, A. and Jacyna, M. (1995) 'The economic and quality of life benefits of helicobacter pylori eradication in chronic duodenal ulcer disease – a community based study', *Post Graduate Medical Journal* 71 (837): 413–18.

Pilpel, D., Leiberman, E., Zadik, Z. and Carel, C. (1995) 'Effect of growth hormone treatment on quality of life of short stature children', *Hormone Research* 44 (1): 1–5.

Porteous, D. (1976) 'Home: the territorial core', *Geographical Review* 66: 383–90.

Rather, M. (1992) 'Nursing as a way of thinking: Heideggerian hermeneutic analysis of the lived experience of the returning RN', *Research in Nursing and Health* 15: 47–55.

Rawles, J. (1989) 'Castigating QALYs', *Journal of Medical Ethics* 15: 143–7.

Rawles, J. and Rawles, K. (1990) 'The QALY argument: a physician's view and a philosopher's view', *Journal of Medical Ethics* 16: 93–4.

Reaves, C. (1992) *Qualitative Research for the Behavioural Sciences*, New York: Wiley.

Relph, E. (1976) *Place and Placelessness*, London: Pion.

Rescher, N. (1972) *Welfare: The Social Issues in Philosophical Perspective*, Pittsburgh, PA: University of Pittsburgh Press.

Ricoeur, P. (1977) 'Schleiermacher's hermeneutics', *Monist* 60: 181–97.

Ricoeur, P. (1981) *Hermeneutics and the Social Sciences*, Cambridge: Cambridge University Press.

Roach, M. and Bubolz-Eicher, J. (1979) 'The language of personal adornment', in J. Cordwell and R. Schwarz (eds) *The Fabrics of Culture: The Anthropology of Clothing and Adornment*, The Hague: Mouton.

Robb, B. (1967) *Sans Everything: A Case to Answer*, London: Nelson.

Rochberg-Halton, E. (1984) 'Object relations, role models, and cultivation of the self', *Environment and Behaviour* 16 (3): 335–68.

Rodin, J. and Langer, E. (1979) 'Long term effects of a control-relevant intervention with the institutionalised aged', *Journal of Personality and Social Psychology* 35: 897–903.

Rodgers, B. and Knafl, K. (1993) *Concept Development in Nursing: Foundations, Techniques and Applications*, Philadelphia, PA: Saunders.

Romney, D., Brown, R. and Fry, P. (1994) 'Improving the quality of life – prescriptions for change', *Social Indicators Research* 33 (1–3): 237–72.

Rowles, D. (1981) 'The surveillance zone as a meaningful space for the aged', *Gerontologist* 21 (3): 304–11.

Rowles, G. (1983a) 'Place and personal identity in old age: observations from Appalachia', *Journal of Environmental Psychology* 3: 299–313.

Rowles, G. (1983b) 'Between worlds: a relocation dilemma for the Appalachian elderly', *International Journal of Aging and Human Development* 17 (4): 301–14.

Roy, C. (1984) *Introduction to Nursing: An Adaptation Model*, 2nd edn, Englewood Cliffs, NJ: Prentice Hall.

Rubinstein, R. (1987) 'The significance of personal objects to older people', *Journal of Aging Studies* 1 (3): 225–38.

Rubinstein, R. (1989) 'The home environments of older people: a description of the psychosocial processes linking person to place', *Journal of Gerontology (Social Sciences)* 44 (2): 45–53.

Rudd, N. (1992) 'Clothing as a signifier in the perceptions of college male homosexuals', *Semiotica* 91 (1/2): 67–78.

Rush, D., Stelmach, W., Young, T., Kirchdorfer, L., Scott Lennox, J., Holverson, H., Sabesin, S. and Nicholas, T. (1995) 'Clinical effectiveness and quality of life with ranitidine vs placebo in gastroesophageal reflux disease patients: a clinical experience network (CEN) study', *Journal of Family Practice* 41 (2): 126–36

Rutman, D. and Freedman, J. (1988) 'Anticipating relocation: coping strategies and the meaning of home for older people', *Canadian Journal on Aging* 7 (1): 17–31.

Schmitt, V., Redondo, J. and Wapner, S. (1977) 'The role of transitional objects in adult adaptation', unpublished manuscript. Available from Seymour Wapner, Heinz Weiner Institute of Developmental Psychology, Clark University, Worcester, MA, 01610, USA.

Schneider, M. (1975) 'Quality of life in large American cities: objective and subjective social indicators', *Social Indicators Research* 1: 495–509.

Seamon, D. (1982) 'The phenomenological contribution to environmental psychology', *Journal of Environmental Psychology* 2: 119–40.

Seashore, S. (1974) 'Measuring the quality of working life', *Social Indicators Research* 1: 135–68.

Seligman, M. (1979) *Erlente Hilflosigkeit* (Learned Helplessness), Munich: Urban and Schwarzenberg.

Sherman, E. and Newman, E. (1977) 'The meaning of cherished personal possessions for the elderly', *Journal of Aging and Human Development* 8 (2): 181–92.

Shin, D. and Johnson, D. (1978) 'Avowed happiness as an overall assessment of quality of life', *Social Indicators Research* 5: 475–92.

Shulz, R. and Brenner, G. (1977) 'Relocation of the aged', *Journal of Gerontology* 32: 323–33.

Singer, P., McKie, J., Kuhse, H. and Richardson, J. (1995) 'Double jeopardy and the use of QALYs in health care allocation', *Journal of Medical Ethics* 21 (3): 144–50.

Stacey, M. (1981) 'The organisation of work in hospital wards', end-of-grant report. SSRC.

Stevenson, L. (1987) *Seven Theories of Human Nature*, 2nd edn, Oxford: Oxford University Press.

Storlie, F. (1982) 'The reshaping of the old', *Journal of Gerontological Nursing* 8 (1): 555–9.

Strabolgi, Lord, Beaumont, Baroness, Heytesbury, Lord, Abel-Smith, B., Ardigonne, E. and Harvey, E. (1965) Letter. *The Times*, 10 November, p. 13.

Strauss, A. (1987) *Qualitative Analysis for Social Scientists*, Cambridge: Cambridge University Press.

Strauss, W., Fortin, T., Hartigan, P., Folland, E. and Parisi, A. (1995) 'A comparison of quality of life scores in patients with angina pectoris after angioplasty compared with after medical therapy: outcomes of a randomized clinical trial', *Circulation* 92 (7): 1710–19.

Sutcliffe, J. and Holmes, S. (1991) 'Quality of life: verification and use of a self-assessment scale in two patient populations', *Journal of Advanced Nursing* 16: 490–8.

Tatarkiewicz, W. (1976) *Analysis of Happiness*, The Hague: Nijhoff.

Taylor, L. and Townsend, A. (1976) 'The local "sense of place" as evidenced in the north of England', *Urban Studies*, 13, 133–46.

Thatcher, M. (1993) *The Downing Street Years*, London: HarperCollins.

Thomas, M. and Lyttle, D. (1980) 'Patient expectations about success of treatment and reported relief from low back pain', *Journal of Psychosomatic Research* 34: 297–301.

Thompson, J. (1981) *Critical Hermeneutics: A Study in the Thought of Paul Ricoeur and Jurgen Habermas*, Cambridge: Cambridge University Press.

Thompson, J. (1991) 'Hermeneutic inquiry', in L. Moody (ed.) *Advancing Nursing Science Through Research*, London: Sage.

Townsend, P. (1962) *The Last Refuge: A Survey of Residential Institutions and Homes for the Aged in England and Wales*, London: Routledge and Kegan Paul.

Tuan, Y. (1977) *Space and Place: The Perspective of Experience*, London: Edward Arnold.

UKCC (1994) *Professional Conduct: Occasional Report on Standards of Nursing Care in Nursing Homes*, London: UKCC.

Veblen, T. (1953) *The Theory of the Leisure Class*, New York: Mentor Books.

Veenhoven, R. (1991) 'Is happiness relative?' *Social Indicators Research* 24: 1–34.

Veenhoven, R. (1994) 'Is happiness a trait?' *Social Indicators Research* 32: 101–60.

Veenhoven, R. (1995) 'World database of happiness', *Social Indicators Research* 34: 299–313.

von Wright, G. (1971) *Explanation and Understanding*, London: Routledge and Kegan Paul.

Wachterhauser, B. (1986) *Hermeneutics and Modern Philosophy*, Albany, NY: State University of New York Press.

Walz, C., Strickland, O. and Lenz, E. (1991) *Measurement in Nursing Research*, 2nd edn, Philadelphia, PA: F. A. Davis.

Wijkstra, P., Ten Vergert, E., van Altena, R., Otten, V., Kraan, J., Postma, D. and Koeter, G. (1995) 'Long term benefits of rehabilitation at home on quality of life and exercise tolerance in patients with chronic obstructive pulmonary disease', *Thorax* 50 (8): 824–8.

Wilkie, R. (1986) 'Basic elements of the concept of individualism', *Philosophical Studies in Education*: 50–63.

Wilkin, D. and Hughes, B. (1987) 'Residential care of elderly people: the consumers' views', *Aging and Society* 7: 125–201.

Willcocks, D., Peace, S. and Kellaher, L. (1987) *Private Lives in Public Places*, London: Tavistock Publications.

Williams, A. (1981) 'Welfare economics and health status measurement', in J. van der Gaag and M. Perlman (eds) *Health, Economics and Health Economics*, Leiden: North Holland.

Williams, A. (1985) 'Economics of coronary artery by-pass grafting', *British Medical Journal* 291: 325–9.

Wilson, B. (1989) (ed.) *About Interpretation: From Plato to Dilthey – A Hermeneutic Anthology*, New York: Lang.

Wilson-Barnett, J. (1980) 'Prevention and alleviation of stress', *Nursing* 10: 432–6.

Winnicott, D. (1951) 'Transitional objects and transitional phenomena', in *D. W Winnicott: Collected Papers* (1958), New York: Basic Books.

Wolk, S. and Telleen, S. (1976) 'Psychological and social correlates of life satisfaction as a function of residential constraint', *Journal of Gerontology* 31 (1): 89–98.

Yin, D., Forman, H. and Langlotz, C. (1995) 'Evaluating health services – the importance of patients' preferences and quality of life', *American Journal of Roentgenology* 165 (6): 1323–8.

Zapf, W. (1984) 'Individual well being – living conditions and perceived quality of life', in W. Glatzer and W. Zapf (eds) *Lebensqualitat in der Bundesrepublik* (*Quality of Life in West Germany*), Munich: Campus.

Zautra, A. and Hempel, A. (1982) 'Subjective well-being and physical health: a narrative literature review with suggestions for future research', *International Journal of Aging and Human Development* 19 (2): 95–10.

# Index